REMEDICALIZING CANNABIS

Intoxicating Histories

Series editors: Virginia Berridge and Erika Dyck

Whether on the street, off the shelf, or over the pharmacy counter, interactions with drugs and alcohol are shaped by contested ideas about addiction, healing, pleasure, and vice and their social dimensions. Books in this series explore how people around the world have consumed, created, traded, and regulated psychoactive substances throughout history. The series connects research on legal and illegal drugs and alcohol with diverse areas of historical inquiry, including the histories of medicine, pharmacy, consumption, trade, law, social policy, and popular culture. Its reach is global and includes scholarship on all periods. Intoxicating Histories aims to link these different pasts as well as to inform the present by providing a firmer grasp on contemporary debates and policy issues. We welcome books, whether scholarly monographs or shorter texts for a broad audience focusing on a particular phenomenon or substance, that alter the state of knowledge.

Remedicalizing Cannabis

Science, Industry, and Drug Policy

SUZANNE TAYLOR

McGill-Queen's University Press
Montreal & Kingston • London • Chicago

ISBN 978-0-2280-1140-8 (cloth)
ISBN 978-0-2280-1349-5 (ePDF)
ISBN 978-0-2280-1350-1 (ePUB)

Legal deposit third quarter 2022
Bibliothèque nationale du Québec

Printed in Canada on acid-free paper that is 100% ancient forest free
(100% post-consumer recycled), processed chlorine free

Library and Archives Canada Cataloguing in Publication

Title: Remedicalizing cannabis : science, industry, and drug policy /
    Suzanne Taylor.
Names: Taylor, Suzanne (Research fellow), author.
Series: Intoxicating histories ; 3.
Description: Series statement: Intoxicating histories ; 3 | Includes bibliographical
    references and index.
Identifiers: Canadiana (print) 20220272263 | Canadiana (ebook) 20220272387 |
    ISBN 9780228011408 (cloth) | ISBN 9780228013495 (ePDF) |
    ISBN 9780228013501 (ePUB)
Subjects: LCSH: Cannabis—Therapeutic use—Great Britain—History—
    20th century. | LCSH: Cannabis—Government policy—Great Britain—
    History—20th century. | LCSH: Marijuana industry—Great Britain—History—
    20th century. | LCSH: Cannabis—Therapeutic use—Great Britain—History—
    21st century. | LCSH: Cannabis—Government policy—Great Britain—History—
    21st century. | LCSH: Marijuana industry—Great Britain—History—21st century.
Classification: LCC RM666.C266 T39 2022 | DDC 615.7/827—dc23

This book was typeset in 10.5/13 New Baskerville ITC Pro.
Copy-editing and composition by T&T Productions Ltd, London.

Contents

Figures

Acknowledgements

This book has been pulled together during lockdown in the time of Covid-19. While separated from my usual networks I note more than ever that this book could not have been written without a most valued team of colleagues, family, and friends.

I especially wish to thank my supervisor, Professor Virginia Berridge, for her efficient supervision, invaluable advice, and support during the PhD, and for her encouragement to turn the latter into a book. I am grateful to my colleagues Dr Stuart Anderson and Dr John Witton for their helpful comments, advice, and encouragement in writing the original PhD; to my examiners Jim Mills and Wayne Hall; to Alex Mold for her help and support; and to all at the Centre for History in Public Health, LSHTM, especially Ingrid James.

This book stems from a Wellcome Trust funded project and I would like to thank the Trust for the opportunity to carry out the research. This was a contemporary history project and I was fortunate to be able to interview those involved in the field. I would like to thank all my interviewees for being so generous with their time and assistance. Archival material has been critical to the project and I thank the library and archival staff at the Wellcome Trust Library, the British Library, the National Archives, the WHO, and the Royal Pharmaceutical Society.

Thanks go to McGill-Queen's University Press for the opportunity to publish; to my editor, Richard Baggaley; and to Sarah Carrington, Sam Clark, and Alex Chambers of T&T Productions for their attention to detail while working on the book.

Huge thanks are also due to friends and family, and particularly to Joy and John for their endless support; to Edward, Tsui-Ling, Lucinda, and Richard for comments and welcome distractions; to James for his red pen and strict adherence to grammar; to Emma for assisting with formatting trauma; to Owen for the food and time; and to Christine, Nicola, and Sumaera for helping me to maintain my sanity.

Abbreviations

ACDD	Advisory Committee on Drug Dependence
ACMD	Advisory Council on the Misuse of Drugs
ACT	Alliance for Cannabis Therapeutics
AIDS	acquired immune deficiency syndrome
ARM	Annual Representative Meeting
BMA	British Medical Association
CAMS	cannabinoids in multiple sclerosis
CANPOP	cannabis for acute post-operative pain
CBD	cannabidiol
CBM	cannabis-based medicine
CBME	cannabis-based medicine extract
CBMP	cannabis-based medical product
CBN	cannabinol
CND	Commission on Narcotic Drugs (United Nations)
CTU	Clinical Trials Unit (Medical Research Council)
CUPID	cannabinoid use in progressive inflammatory brain disease
DDA	Dangerous Drugs Act
DDT	dichlorodiphenyltrichloroethane
DHSS	Department of Health and Social Security
ECRS	endogenous cannabinoid receptor system
EGEC	Expert Group on the Effects of Cannabis
FDA	Food and Drug Administration (United States)
HODI	Home Office Drugs Inspectorate

ICI	Imperial Chemical Industries
INCB	International Narcotics Control Board
INDP	Investigative New Drugs Programme
IOP	intraocular pressure
LCC	Legalise Cannabis Campaign
LSD	lysergic acid diethylamide
MCA	Medicines Control Agency
MDA	Misuse of Drugs Act
MHRA	Medicines and Healthcare products Regulatory Agency
MOA	mechanism of action
MP	Member of Parliament
MRC	Medical Research Council
MS	multiple sclerosis
NCE	new chemical entity
NHS	National Health Service
NIDA	National Institute on Drug Abuse
NIH	National Institutes of Health
NIHR	National Institute for Health and Care Research
NIMH	National Institute of Mental Health
PLR	'product licence of right'
RCT	randomized controlled trial
RPS	Royal Pharmaceutical Society
SOMA	Society of Mental Awareness
THC	tetrahydrocannabinol
UN	United Nations
UNODC	United Nations Office on Drugs and Crime
WGC	Working Group on Cannabis
WHO	World Health Organization

REMEDICALIZING CANNABIS

Introduction

A DANGEROUS MEDICINE

The use of cannabis as a medicine has a history stretching back to ancient times, but in the twentieth century it was caught up in prohibitive international legislation, becoming regulated solely as an illicit drug by 1973. Yet, almost as soon as it lost its legal status as a medicine, it began undergoing a process of remedicalization. The United Kingdom was at the forefront of early research on cannabis, helping to expand our knowledge of its pharmacology and later developing cannabis-based medicinal products (CBMPs). Cannabis reappeared in different therapeutic forms for a range of uses, including as an anti-emetic for chemotherapy-related nausea, as an appetite stimulant to combat wasting due to acquired immune deficiency syndrome (AIDS), as an anti-glaucoma agent, as an asthma relief agent, as an analgesic, and as an agent for the relief of neurological disorders such as epilepsy and multiple sclerosis (MS). These drugs were used infrequently and had numerous problems, not least their placement in the most restrictive Schedules of drug control systems, so patient pressure drove demand for alternative products.

In its botanical form cannabis appeared to offer a more effective way forward for patients who self-medicated. A biotechnology pharmaceutical firm – a small UK start-up – was established in 1998 specifically to look into herbal cannabis. It developed a cannabis-based medicine (CBM) called Sativex that included extracts of cannabis that would be administered orally as a spray for the treatment of spasticity in MS. Thus, with cannabis's twin roles (as licit medicine and illicit drug) reinstated, the concept of cannabis therapeutics became tied up with drug control discussions. It appeared that the policy environment around cannabis had shifted when it was downgraded to class C in the drug Schedules in 2004. At this point it seemed that cannabis was moving in line with opium and morphine, in that it could legitimately exist in both controlled illicit drug and licit medical structures. By 2020 the United Kingdom had become one of the world's biggest providers of CBMPs.

Yet, the fact that both licit medical avenues and illicit recreational channels existed for cannabis left it operating as a borderline substance within drug control mechanisms. In the United Kingdom the confusion around cannabis's position has led to rapid policy shifts that fail to satisfy anyone: not members of parliament (MPs) or patients, not policymakers, regulators, industry experts, or scientists. There exists a paradoxical situation in the United Kingdom, where, despite the country being a big producer of CBMPs, UK patients have very limited access to those products. Patients contend that this is because access is hindered by regulation and that CBMPs are available only for arbitrarily determined diseases. Sativex, for example, was never widely available in the United Kingdom and was not recommended by the National Health Service (NHS) for certain conditions until 2019. Since 2017, headline-grabbing news items showing seriously ill children being refused cannabis treatment or their parents being forced to buy prohibitively expensive medicines caused a public outcry, and it meant that rapid policy shifts have taken place to ameliorate the situation in the United Kingdom.

The problem does not exist only at a national level: it also poses a huge headache internationally. Countries have been providing access to CBMPs via a variety of mechanisms. Pharmaceutical CBMPs are available on prescription in the United Kingdom, but provision is very limited and expensive. The Netherlands, in comparison, allows herbal or non-pharmaceutical preparations. Some countries, including Canada and Uruguay, have legalized cannabis for medicinal or even recreational purposes, while access in others remains strictly controlled. Potter and Weinstock's edited collection explores cannabis legalization in Canada.[1] Even the provision of legal medical cannabis can cause problems, and research has shown how the legalization of cannabis has the potential to disadvantage medical users, as the interests of companies shift to the more extensive recreational market.

International policy has struggled to keep up. The World Health Organization (WHO) argued in the 1950s that there was no justification for medical use, but by 2018 it was recommending the removal of cannabis extracts, tinctures, and preparations from international control regimes.[2] The International Narcotics Control Board (INCB), previously very wary of the medical cannabis movement, stated in 2019 that it does not prohibit medicinal cannabis provided that countries comply with the relevant treaties.[3] In 2020, acting on WHO recommendations, the United Nations (UN) Commission on Narcotic Drugs (CND) reclassified cannabis and cannabis resin under an international listing that recognized their medical value. Cannabis, whether for recreational or medical use, is no longer a fringe product – it is potentially big business. The lines are increasingly blurred between medical and recreational uses, and there is growing pressure from international firms to gain access to the potentially lucrative markets involved. In the United Kingdom, division between the NHS and private provision further complicates policy positions. How we regulate cannabis and its derivatives is a conundrum that is drawing in patients, policymakers, industries, and consumers.[4]

Framed as a history of science and policymaking, this book provides an account of the intersection of science, industry, activism, and policy – a dynamic space in which the process of remedicalization has unfolded. Sociologists have investigated the concept of medicalization in relation to people and disease, but it can be extended to products: in this case, cannabis.[5] I use the term 'remedicalization' as opposed to 'medicalization' because cannabis had a licit medical past prior to 1973. I define remedicalization as the reintroduction of medical uses and structures of the drug, as distinct from nonmedical illicit uses and control structures. This book recognizes that full remedicalization has not yet been established, instead examining the intervening stages of that transition: from research, through product development and clinical trials to regulation. In considering what kind of 'borderline substance' cannabis has become (the regulatory term used for tobacco, discussed in the next section), I explore the process whereby boundaries have shifted between illicit 'drug' and licit 'medicine'. To what extent has cannabis been remedicalized? How did this process take place? How has remedicalization been incorporated in the drug policy structures, and what impact has medicalization had on these mechanisms?

This book focuses primarily on the United Kingdom, although some account is given of different national contexts. The emphasis is on the period from 1973, when cannabis was dropped as a medicine in the United Kingdom, to 2004, when cannabis was

downgraded to class C. This research does, however, take account
of developments prior to 1973 that enabled research in the 1970s to
take off, as well as important developments that occurred after the
main period of interest, up to 2020.

National and international debates over cannabis and drug control mechanisms are contentious and divisive. A clear understanding
of the history of the medicinal use of cannabis is important. Throw-
ing light on science–policy transfer is relevant beyond cannabis as
we see increasing debate over the use and positioning of other potential medicinal drugs, such as psilocybin, and other 'intoxicating
substances' along the spectrum, including alcohol, tobacco, and
coffee. But it is also of broader importance in helping to guide policy in relation to other public health topics, ranging from obesity to
pollution and pandemics.

THE UNDERSTANDING OF CANNABIS ACROSS TIME AND PLACE

There exists a myriad of books on cannabis. Increased recreational
drug use in the 1960s and increasingly prohibitive legislation attracted much historical research. Academic historical work focused
on the long-term history of the drug's use in many parts of the world
and also on how perspectives on substances fluctuate over time and
place.[6] Ernest Abel has shown that cannabis was not always viewed
as an illicit, dangerous substance but was initially prized as a food,
fibre, and medicine.[7] Theodore Brunner has analysed literary evidence to demonstrate cannabis use in ancient Greece and Rome.[8]
The reinvestigation of old literature in the light of contemporary
knowledge and the identification of similarities between contemporary and historical concerns over issues such as toxicity, delivery
methods, and dosage have been other facets of historical research.[9]
Lewis has highlighted how debates and fears generated in the 1960s
over drugs such as cannabis and heroin bore a striking resemblance
to those generated in the nineteenth century.[10] David Soloman edited a collection of essays in 1969 on the historical, sociological,
and cultural aspects of cannabis, in which he argued for its legalization.[11] Other works, such as those by Matthews or Booth, centre on
'cannabis culture' in the United States or the United Kingdom and
concentrate on the legalization versus prohibition axis of the debate.[12] This book, while taking recreational arguments into account,

focuses on the medical aspects of the debate, though it does consider the impact of remedicalization on regulation and, likewise, the implication of restrictions on the development of cannabis as a medicine.

In answering the aforementioned questions about the process of remedicalization, we must look beyond the literature on cannabis itself and illicit drugs in general. Two concepts are useful: firstly, cannabis as a 'borderline substance'; and secondly, cannabis as a plant in the context of the rise of phytopharmacy.

Peculiar or borderline substances

Over the period studied in this book, cannabis was viewed as a 'peculiar' or 'borderline' substance, one whose position as a medical and/or recreational product was fluid and dependent on a myriad of developing and competing factors. Star and Griesemer, in a historical study of the University of California's Museum of Vertebrate Zoology in Berkeley, introduced the concept of 'boundary objects' in relation to records or documents, and they showed how different groups – such as amateur collectors, professional scientists, and administrators – gave different interpretations of the same sources. 'Boundary objects' were able to bridge the gaps between the different understandings and goals of the different groups.[13]

This concept of boundary objects has been adopted for many different situations. In the medical history field, it was adopted by Epstein in relation to AIDS.[14] Epstein also showed, in his study of the relationship between activism and science, that a virus or a medication could be a boundary object, but, in essence, the object was one that could cross social networks, having a subtle but significantly different meaning depending on where it was viewed from.

Berridge, in her study of the shifting understanding of substances, focused on opiates and tobacco to show how the boundary between licit and illicit is a shifting and negotiable one.[15] She showed how substances such as tobacco could be portrayed as having an indeterminate nature: was it a food, a medicine, or a drug?[16] She considered 'altered states' or 'the cultural and policy milieu' in which drugs are regulated, as well as the social and political factors that drive change.[17]

Sherratt, writing on the history of narcotics and stimulants, analysed how we define drugs, particularly psychoactive substances, and viewed cannabis as one of a group of 'peculiar substances' that can cross the line from being a widely consumed substance to a dangerous drug.[18] Goode took a sociological approach to looking at why we have controversies around these substances, investigating the impact of bias. He argued that the controversy over cannabis was due to political, not scientific, debate and was more a result of previously held ideological commitments than of any new scientific arguments.[19] Ungerleider and Andrysiak's work on bias and the cannabis researcher showed how chemicals were seen as moral as well as pharmacological substances.[20] Cannabis thus has a fluid and ever-changing position across time and space. This raises questions about what the process is whereby boundaries shift between 'drug' and 'medicine,' and what the issues and interests involved in that transaction are.

Cannabis as a plant: the rise of phytomedicine

Cannabis, which is often viewed solely as an illicit drug, must instead be viewed as a plant; the revival of its use as a therapeutic needs to be considered within the context of the revival of plant-based medicine.[21] Historical research on medicinal plants has concentrated on three aspects. Firstly, there are the histories of the disciplines of botany and herbalism. Works generally centre on the early history of botany and herbals, particularly in the Middle Ages.[22] Those who have looked at 'medical history from below' have stressed the nineteenth-century popular interest in medical botany and its subsequent commercial development.[23] Secondly, a more recent trend has been the study of the development of ethnobotany: that is, the study of medicinal plants and indigenous knowledge.[24] And thirdly, there are the histories of individual plants.[25]

The discovery of *Artemisia annua* (*A. annua*) inspired a number of thought-provoking, short pieces of historical writing, including Dobson's examination of quinine and artemisinin.[26] Power's study of drug resistance looked briefly at the history of *A. annua*'s discovery and use, viewing its acceptance in terms of 'contested knowledge'.[27] Goodman and Walsh's study of Taxol (paclitaxel) traced the 'cultural biography' through which a plant became a commercial product.[28] The rise of these disciplines is important for understanding the process of developing drugs from a plant. A witness seminar on 'Drugs in Psychiatric Practice', organized by the Wellcome Trust in 1998, and Healy's book *The Creation of Psychopharmacology* have both traced the development of psychopharmacology, and in particular they have looked at the role of industry, the rise of the 'magic bullet' approach, the importance of standardization, and the tensions between disciplines.[29] Russo has argued that Europeans were important for the development of cannabis-based drugs, as, despite the US National Institute on Drug Abuse (NIDA) providing the majority of funding into cannabis research and introducing CBM, Europeans had not 'strayed quite so far from the realm of *materia medica*'.[30]

Many of the debates about plant medicine are transferable to an investigation of cannabis, and they allow the medical use of cannabis to be viewed in the broader context of the development of phytopharmacy. The myriad constituents found in cannabis, as in any plant, posed problems in early research, but in later years they looked to be a key benefit for therapeutics. The desire to create a medicine out of herbal cannabis created heated debate over which form would be researched, developed, and licensed. Deciding which aspects of a plant we consider to be a medicine (the whole plant, extracts like tetrahydrocannabinol (THC), or synthetic versions, used singularly or in combination) and who makes that call or has 'ownership' is fundamental and inescapable in drug scheduling debates. These previous works on the history of other plant-based drugs show that we must ask about the ways in which current policy debates on cannabis are related not to its position as an illicit drug but to its existence as a plant-based medicine.

Within this broader context, in order to understand the process of remedicalization that cannabis is undergoing, I explore issues and interest involved in that transition, including scientific knowledge and disciplines, science–policy exchange, industry, lay knowledge and patient activism, and evidence-based medicine through the mechanism of clinical trials.

Changing scientific knowledge

Changing scientific knowledge has been critical in the remedicalization of cannabis. Cannabis had a long medicinal history before its removal from the United Kingdom's medical scene in 1973, so it is worth reflecting on the history of, and knowledge about, cannabis prior to that date.

Cannabis was introduced to the United Kingdom as a medical product in the nineteenth century. Berridge's work highlights cannabis's shifting role from 'wonder drug' to sidelined substance.[31] Berridge has described its introduction to the United Kingdom as a therapeutic in the 1840s by William O'Shaughnessy, an Irish doctor, who served as a professor of chemistry and medicine in the Medical College in Calcutta, India.[32] O'Shaughnessy wrote about its analgesic and sedative properties, finding major success in treating both muscle spasm, caused by tetanus or rabies, and vomiting from cholera. His work attracted considerable attention because these diseases were much feared at the time.

This raises interesting questions over which diseases have been important in the remedicalization of cannabis – and why. History demonstrates that changing scientific knowledge and technology have allowed commercial success, such as when the pharmacist Peter Squire produced a cannabis extract that became readily available for many ailments. Official recognition was achieved and quality standards were set when CBMS were included in UK and US pharmacopoeias in the 1850s.[33] The development of Squire's extract was important, because the medicinal value of a plant was linked to its 'active principle' rather than to the plant itself.[34] Numerous alkaloids were isolated in pure form – for instance, morphine was purified and medicalized from the poppy – but cannabis was disadvantaged because, while alkaloids were relatively easy to isolate, isolating cannabinoids from cannabis proved more difficult.

The value of cannabis as a medicine only increased in the 1890s when the chemists Wood, Spivey, and Easterfield, at Cambridge University, succeeded in obtaining a relatively pure extraction of a terpene, which was thought to be the active principle of cannabis and which they called cannabinol (CBN). This discovery facilitated research on its use as an antibiotic, an appetite stimulant, and an antidepressant, as well as its use to treat opium addiction. Smoking was recommended as the fastest and most effective method of delivery.

Despite these advances, cannabis quickly fell out of favour. Berridge has offered explanations for this: uncertainty of action, irregular supply, and the drug's inability to compete with opium products in terms of availability and mode of delivery.[35] The pure active principle had not been isolated, which was a major problem at a time when the pharmaceutical sector was developing around the production of single chemical entities. Its chemical structure meant that it was not water soluble, unlike morphine (a major competitor). Consequently, cannabis could not be administered via new

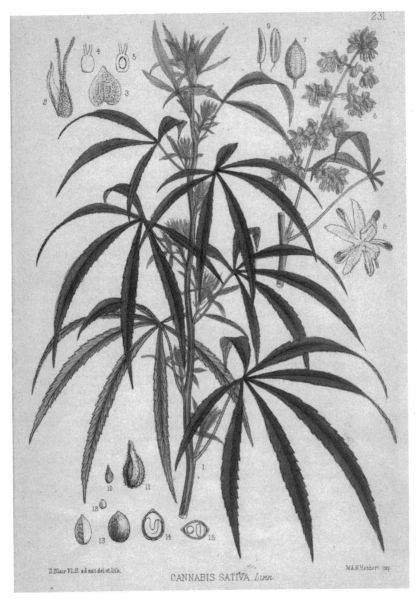

Figure 0.1   *Cannabis sativa*, Linn.

drug-delivery systems such as the hypodermic syringe, which was rapidly gaining currency. Issues of standardization posed further complications, as there was no standard for either the total content of cannabinoids or the proportions of individual cannabinoids, leaving the product in a weakened position compared with emergent synthetic single chemical entities such as aspirin. All these factors limited cannabis's utility as a therapeutic in a marketplace increasingly controlled by the developing pharmaceutical industry.

Did overcoming the problems faced in the nineteenth century allow the process of remedicalization to take off? Post-1973 this book explores how the rise of new disciplines like psychopharmacology, clinical pharmacology, and the work of chemists and pharmacologists rapidly expanded our knowledge of cannabis. The isolation of the active compounds, the discovery of cannabis's mode of action, improved supply and standardization, and new delivery systems all opened the door to research and medical applications.

Safety and harm relative to other drugs

Cannabis's safety and harms in comparison with other drugs are continual elements of debate today. Pre-empting controversial contemporary comparisons with other drugs, Walter Ernest Dixon – a leading member of the United Kingdom's Rolleston Committee on Morphine and Heroin Addiction in the 1920s and an opponent of the penal narcotic policy in the American model – placed cannabis in the same category as tea and coffee rather than alongside drugs such as heroin. At this stage, cannabis was generally regarded as a safe medicine: CBMs such as cannabis tinctures were available as over-the-counter products, and cannabis extracts were found in many proprietary medicines – they were often combined with opium and capsicum extracts as a painkiller.[36]

But in the nineteenth century cannabis use had increasingly been linked to mental health problems, especially insanity, and to crime. Much of the evidence for this had come from India, where it was feared that hospitals were full of patients with mental health problems that were allegedly caused by cannabis use. A major inquiry by the Indian Hemp Drugs Commission of the 1890s examined the trade in hemp drugs and whether cannabis use should be prohibited. The commission concluded that there was no link between cannabis and crime and no need for prohibition. But the alleged connection to mental health problems became a recurring theme in cannabis debates. Though the commission's report was largely ignored in the United Kingdom at the time, it became of interest to historians and scientists from the 1970s onwards. Kalant, for example, reviewed the report and reflected on its relevance to contemporary problems.[37]

Interest in the mental health aspects re-emerged from 2000 onwards, and debates over the alleged link were revived, most notably by British psychiatrists. Basu has discussed the evidence from the Hemp Drugs Commission for the link to insanity,[38] while Mills has worked on the growth of lunatic asylums in India in the nineteenth century and placed cannabis within the colonial discussions of madness, also considering the impact of these discussions on UK discourse.[39] Guba explored cannabis in nineteenth-century France and the impact of the French Empire.[40] The possible link between cannabis and mental health problems remains hotly debated and has operated as something of a countervailing force to remedicalization. Fears over the harms of cannabis in relation to mental health resulted in a hardening of attitudes among policymakers, leading the drug to be reclassified as class B again in 2009. Questions over cannabis harms in relation to the harms of other drugs have proved critical in its positioning in drug control systems, and they have at times hindered medical research and patient access.

The reintroduction of cannabis's dual function as a borderline substance used for both recreational and medicinal purposes shook drug control systems. When the psychiatrists Griffith Edwards and John Strang used the headline 'Britain's Drugs Crisis: Recipe for Dangerous Medicine'[41] in 1994 to make their case for the maintenance of the drug control system and to emphasize the dangers of drug legalization, the phrase could also be applied to cannabis in its role as a therapeutic within the UK drug control framework. The rapid fluctuations of cannabis's position as a borderline drug drew attention to the validity or otherwise of the UK control system. Cannabis remained a 'dangerous medicine', and cannabis harms included its threat to the stability or structure of the control framework. There were calls for the entire system to be re-evaluated, and comparisons were drawn between cannabis and licit drugs such as alcohol and tobacco.

International drug control mechanisms and international agencies

Policy history is a major strand of cannabis literature. In the twentieth century cannabis became increasingly tied up in the development of prohibitive policy. However, much of the historical work is US-centric, with an emphasis on the period before 1945, looking, for example, at the prohibitive American drug control policies of the 1930s. These were implemented via the Marijuana (Cannabis) Tax Act of 1937 through the Federal Bureau of Narcotics, which was headed by Harry Anslinger.[42] Saper has suggested that American narcotic laws had developed more through accident and the acceptance of drug myths rather than through rational decision-making.[43] More recently, Jim Mills has looked at controls and consumption in the United Kingdom, expanding our knowledge of colonial production and supply, as well as the development of initial prohibitive international and domestic legislation.[44] He has demonstrated how the politics of empire led to prohibitive drug policies, while scientific evaluation was pushed to the sidelines in favour of the demands of supply and trade. Mills revealed the battle between the producer and the trader and looked at how producers sought to avoid tax imposed by the British administration, which led to cannabis becoming associated with crime in the eyes of the British government. In domestic policy he demonstrated how policy seemed to be formed by misunderstandings.

Whatever the reasons behind policy changes were, they had a significant impact on cannabis's position as a medicine. When the WHO declared in 1952 that 'cannabis preparations are practically obsolete' and added that 'there is no justification for the medical use of cannabis preparations,'[45] it seemed that the drug's long career as a medicine was over.[46] With no accepted medical use, cannabis then became viewed mainly as a drug of misuse, as regulation around medical and recreational drugs was tightened.

In 1961 cannabis fell under the control of the UN Single Convention on Narcotic Drugs. The Single Convention introduced four Schedules into which drugs were classified, with Schedule I and Schedule IV being the most stringent. These Schedules controlled the use of these drugs based on their therapeutic value and the risk of abuse.

- Schedule I contains substances with addictive properties, presenting a serious risk of abuse. It includes cannabis and its derivatives, cocaine, heroin, methadone, morphine, and opium.
- Schedule II contains substances normally used for medical purposes and presenting the lowest risk of abuse.
- Schedule III contains preparations of substances listed in Schedule II, as well as preparations of cocaine.

- Schedule IV is the Schedule with the strictest level of control, and it includes the most dangerous substances already listed in Schedule I that are of extremely limited medical or therapeutic value. It includes cannabis, cannabis resin, and heroin.

Cannabis and cannabis resin along with heroin were listed in both Schedule I and Schedule IV, which entitled parties to adopt 'special measures of control', and to ban the substances altogether apart from in medical or scientific research. Cannabis in the form of extracts or tinctures was placed in the slightly less restrictive Schedule I, alongside morphine.

Bewley has written on the evolution of drug control, such as the development of the Single Convention on Narcotic Drugs, and Bruun has examined the Nordic experience of controlling medicines and of international drug control after World War II.[47] The structure of regulatory frameworks has been analysed by McAllister. He considered the involvement of various interests in policy formation: colonial concerns, pharmaceutical interests, and the role of interpersonal relationships. Of particular interest is his discussion of the development of a split between the licit medical use and the illicit recreational use of drugs in the West – a divide that cannabis appeared to straddle.[48] He drew attention to divergences between precautionary, paternalistic approaches and liberal principles. This aspect played a critical role in debates between key pharmacologists and in policy discussions on the medical applications of cannabis in the United Kingdom.

In 1971 the UN Convention on Psychotropic Substances consolidated previous legislation and incorporated emergent synthetic psychotropic drugs into the Schedules that are not covered in the Single Convention. Cannabis-based drugs were placed in Schedule I, which included substances that had no, or very limited, medical value. Cannabis itself remained controlled under the Single Convention.

- Schedule I contains substances presenting a high risk of abuse, posing a particularly serious threat to public health, and having very little or no therapeutic value. The level of control is very strict: use is prohibited except for scientific or limited medical purposes. This Schedule includes LSD, MDMA (ecstasy), mescaline, psilocybin, and tetrahydrocannabinol (THC).

- Schedule II contains substances presenting a risk of abuse, posing a serious threat to public health, which are of low or moderate therapeutic value.
- Schedule III contains substances presenting a risk of abuse, posing a serious threat to public health, which are of moderate or high therapeutic value.
- Schedule IV contains substances presenting a risk of abuse, posing a minor threat to public health, with a high therapeutic value. These are available for therapeutic purposes. This Schedule includes tranquillizers, analgesics, and narcotics, such as allobarbital, diazepam, lorazepam, phenobarbital, and temazepam.

These conventions were open to interpretation, and different parties adopted different approaches to drug control. The US domestic legislation, for example, excluded medical use of substances listed in Schedule I from their domestic Controlled Substances Act, although the international conventions permitted limited use. These conventions were important because they excluded cannabis as a medicine, which had a significant legal impact back in the United Kingdom.

UK domestic drug control policy

The United Kingdom ratified the Single Convention in 1964, when the Drugs (Prevention of Misuse) Act enacted the provisions necessary for compliance and made the cultivation of cannabis an offence. This was succeeded by subsequent Dangerous Drugs Acts (DDAS), such as the DDA of 1965, which consolidated previous acts, and the DDA of 1967, which introduced the stop and search policy. Many drugs had dual structures, and drugs covered by the acts could be made available as medicines, since there existed some overlap between controlled illicit drugs and regulated medicines.

Cannabis as a medicine was still permissible in the 1960s, and when the 1968 Medicines Act was introduced, extracts of cannabis, in the form of tinctures, were made available on prescription via a 'product licence of right' (PLR). In the 1970s, however, cannabis lost its dual structure. The Misuse of Drugs Act (MDA) was enacted in 1971 in the United Kingdom, introducing the term 'controlled drugs'. The main purpose of the Act was to prevent the misuse of controlled drugs, and to do this it imposed a complete ban on the

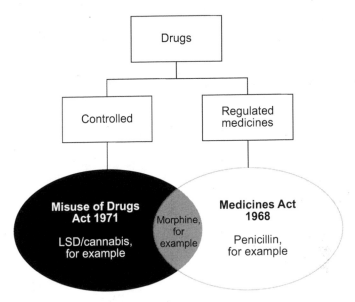

Figure 0.2   Regulation of drugs.

possession, supply, manufacture, import, and export of controlled drugs except as allowed by regulations or by a licence from the Secretary of State. The Act also introduced the Advisory Council on the Misuse of Drugs (ACMD), a statutory body that would advise the government. Schedule II of the Act identified the drugs that were to be controlled, dividing them into three classes: A, B, and C. The level of classification determined the severity of penalties that could be imposed under criminal law for an infringement of the Act. Drugs derived from cannabis, e.g. cannabinoids such as CBD and delta-9-THC, were placed in class A. Cannabis and cannabis resin were listed as class B, which enabled cannabis to be used under licence from the Home Office for research purposes, or for clinical trials with permission from the Medicines Control Agency (MCA). But over time cannabis's position within the classes would fluctuate; for example, in 2004 cannabis was reclassified to class C, and it then went back to class B in 2009. Regulations in the Act permitted exemptions for legitimate activities such as the medical use of controlled drugs, but the last remaining cannabis product, tinctures, was banned when these came into force. When the 'product licences of right' were reviewed by the MCA, cannabis's licence was not renewed; when the original regulations of the MDA were then enacted in 1973, cannabis resin and CBN and its derivatives were placed in Schedule IV – which comprised substances with no known, or limited, medical use – and were therefore not exempted under the regulations. Cannabis, in any form, could no longer be prescribed and was left under the sole control of illicit drug regulations.[49]

At face value these moves could have ended cannabis's career as a medical drug, but the removal of CBM from the medicine cabinet was perhaps just a hiatus in the plant's history: even as it was removed, cannabis was beginning its comeback as a licit medicine, and CBM rapidly re-entered the clinic, first in synthetic form and later as extracts.

Science–policy transfer and the role of expert advice

In the United Kingdom the framing of cannabis and its derivatives in drug policy has been reviewed by expert governmental bodies. Discussions include both the closed in-house reviews by the ACMD and the more public discussions that emerged in the 1990s through the House of Lords Science and Technology Committee and professional bodies such as the British Medical Association (BMA), all of which published influential reports on the medical use of cannabis.

Historical and social science work from the wider literature provides methods of looking at the role of expert advice that can be applied to the cannabis field. The term 'expert advice' covers a variety of structures, as Barker and Peters describe, ranging from institutional expert civil servants and advisory committees to more informal information networks and contacts.[50] In the UK context, MacLeod has shown how the roles of the professional and the expert developed in the mid-Victorian period, while Hamlin has described how disputes between these specialists flared up.[51] Expert advice evolved into a more formalized setting in the twentieth century, and Berridge discussed the development of advisory bodies or expert committees in her analysis of smoking policy in Britain. She placed deliberations over smoking in the context of the developing relationships between experts and the state and of the growing demand for the 'rational expertise-based model' within government, especially within the context of health policy and developments in the NHS. As Berridge showed, the model of channelling scientific advice into policy was utilized in the illicit drugs field, and the formula was developed in detail during the 1970s, with the formation of the ACMD.[52] It was during the 1960s that some of the initial expert committees in the illicit drugs field were established, on an ad hoc basis, and then the 1970s saw the formation of statutory committees, which became deeply concerned with the cannabis question.

The formal structure of an expert committee may be seen as one of the better routes to achieving evidence-based policy. Bulmer showed how it provides a method of neutralizing a subject by taking it out of the political arena.[53] This is especially important for a highly divisive issue such as cannabis. To what extent a committee can be successful in this is open to question, though. Covid-19 has clearly demonstrated the peril of science–policy transfer in the face of uncertainty. Jasanoff, for example, in looking at the role of expert committees in discussing carcinogens in the United States in the 1970s and 1980s, found that they were increasingly important to policymakers, and she illustrated how the technocratic model is by no means value-free. Her work considered what lies behind the construction of 'evidence' or expert advice. Jasanoff demonstrated how 'scientific uncertainty is a resource that can be mobilized by regulators … in effect to influence policy'.

In the case of cannabis, uncertainty over its medical benefits and potential hazards was utilized by those on both sides of the debate. Hilgartner, reviewing expert advice in relation to diet and cancer, demonstrated how uncertainty could be invoked to justify action or inaction. He also raised another issue: the role of private/public discussions. Information leaks blurred the division between this public and private space. This portrayal is useful in the case of cannabis, where uncertainty, conflict, and leaks played key roles in the expert discussions. Florin, in a review of the relationship between science and policy in the area of coronary heart disease prevention, found that high levels of scientific uncertainty led to different interpretations of the evidence by those coming from different backgrounds. This was a problem in areas that lacked an independent system such as an expert committee.

The role of professional bodies and expert committees has been studied relatively little in relation to cannabis, even though rich archival material exists. I show how expert groups proved critical by providing an area for discussion of medical cannabis and by stimulating clinical trials, involving industry, and later by re-evaluating

questions of access; it is also interesting to examine how they ne-
gotiated questions of uncertainty. They have not been without
controversy though, which has led to debates over the mechanism
of science–policy transfer, independence, and transparency.

Lay knowledge and patient activism

The increasing use of cannabis in the 1960s, because of its availability as a plant, meant that, unlike with most drugs, lay knowledge of
its medical properties existed long before the prohibitive legislation
was introduced and before it became a pharmaceutically produced
product. Despite increased controls on drugs, there remained widespread illicit access to cannabis, and a battle over the 'ownership' of
cannabis emerged. Lay knowledge and patient activism thus proved
to be key components in remedicalization.

Patient activism has been examined in relation to diseases such as
MS and AIDS.[54] Mold has examined patients as consumers.[55] Literature has also looked at the role of illicit cannabis growers.[56] Patient
experience of cannabis has been studied but with a focus on the
United States. For example, Randall provided a personal account of
his experience with cannabis and glaucoma in the United States and
discussed the development of the legal defence termed 'medical
necessity'.[57] Dufton provided a historical account of lay knowledge
and legalization activism in the United States, in which medical aspects played a part.[58] Bock looked at the politics of medical cannabis
in the United States,[59] and Newhart and Dolphin provided a sociological examination of the US patient experience with cannabis,
looking at obstacles to medicalization, including stigma and legal
hindrances.[60] Scholarship points to a shift from activism to partnerships, with patients as policy actors.

Little has been written about the UK patient experience. In the
United Kingdom, patient activism by MS patients was a key driver in
the process of remedicalization, forcing consideration of the need
for additional medicines and clinical trials and shaping the research
that took place. The perceived 'respectability' of these MS patient
conferred legitimacy on stigmatized products, and their ability to
forge strong relationships between doctors, patients, industry, and
policymakers drove – and continues to drive – the process of remedicalization. But once CBMPs were again being produced, few
patients found that they could access the drugs; in more recent

years, activism has brought the question of access, particularly free access on the NHS rather than via private provision, to the fore, forcing rapid policy change.

The role of the pharmaceutical industry

In the twentieth century, the history of therapeutics is inseparable from the rise of the pharmaceutical industry. Since the 1990s industry has become an important location for research into new cannabis products. McAllister has demonstrated the role played by interest groups such as the pharmaceutical industry in the formation of drug control mechanisms. He demonstrated how the 1961 UN Single Convention on Narcotic Drugs favoured a medical–industrial complex, focusing on how control of the raw material affected the producer rather than the control of new synthetic derivatives, an exclusion which largely continued in the 1970s.

Historical literature on the role of industry in the remedicalization of cannabis in the twentieth century, especially in the UK context, is nevertheless limited. That which does exist focuses on the development of synthetic products, such as nabilone in the United States, rather than on the development of the herbal product, which has been the focus of UK industry. A number of studies have looked at the long history of therapeutics, highlighting the brevity of synthetic drug usage, as opposed to a long, herbal tradition. The influence of factors such as regulatory processes and scientific advances in drug development has attracted attention.[61] Pickstone has traced the growing intersection of industrial and scientific interest in the interwar years, while others have focused on developments in the pharmaceutical industry in the immediate post-war years – a time of great optimism surrounding the advent of new drug treatments.[62]

The changing focus from infectious to chronic disease in the pharmaceutical industry has attracted attention, as have research flows between countries and their impact on industry.[63] In the initial development of the pharmaceutical industry, historians cite the importance of a greater understanding of vegetable and mineral substances used as medicine.[64] In this research, the isolation of an active principle was important. Major discoveries included the isolation of morphine from opium, aspirin from willow bark, and later quinine from cinchona. Authors writing about the pharmaceutical

industry and about pharmacy as a scientific discipline have highlighted the importance of access to research material and how it can
shape social and cognitive developments. Histories of pharmacy and
the pharmaceutical industry divide their development into between
three and five stages: kitchen physic; the rise of commercial remedies; the development of pathology and microbiology; the growth
of multinational pharmaceutical companies, acquisitions and mergers, and the elimination of small-scale industry; and the emergence
of small biotechnology companies.

After 1973 the role of the pharmaceutical industry was fundamental in the remedicalization of cannabis in the United Kingdom. The
creation of a UK biotechnology firm producing plant-based medicinal cannabis products provides an interesting case study, covering
the role of the pharmaceutical industry, supply, standardization,
and patient activism. The United Kingdom has especially focused
on the provision of a pharmaceutical-based product as a mechanism
for splitting recreational arguments from medical ones. In his book
*White Market Drugs: Big Pharma and the Hidden History of Addiction
in America*, Hertzog wrote that there was perhaps a false dichotomy
between legitimate pharmaceutical product and dangerous illicit
drug, and that decisions over regulation had more to do with respectability than the pharmacological understanding of harms.[65]

One feature of the medical history of cannabis has been the publication of histories by the scientists involved in reinvestigating the
drug. In the United States, Mikuriya, a former director of marijuana
research for the National Institute of Mental Health (NIMH) and
consultant to the National Commission on Marihuana and Drug
Abuse, wrote in the mid-1970s of people's amnesia about cannabis's
original uses.[66] Several industry histories have emerged since the
2000s, such as that by Russo, senior medical adviser to GW Pharmaceuticals, who provided a short history of cannabis's medical role.
There is, nevertheless, limited independent historical discussion of
the remedicalization that has taken place post-1973.[67]

Bias and the role of history

As a final point it is important to note that the 'history' of cannabis has been co-opted to support contemporary arguments for and
against the use of cannabis. The presumed relationship between
cannabis, violence, and crime – an argument pushed by Henry

Anslinger, the first head of the Federal Narcotics Control Board in the United States – was given support by the supposed use of cannabis by the Assassins, a sect of Shia Muslims who were alleged to have taken cannabis prior to assassination attempts. Casto has challenged the view that history can be used in such a manner to support policy, and he has attempted to debunk the Assassins tale as a myth.[68] More recent material by Berridge has also considered the relationship between history and policy, challenging the assumption of Queen Victoria's use of cannabis for dysmenorrhoea and its utilization in policy debate.[69] Cannabis is tied up in a loaded history. Understanding the history of cannabis can help us understand the path of cannabis medicines, the discrepancy between emergent cannabis drugs and patient demands, science–policy transfer, and the rapid fluctuations in policy seen around the world.

CHAPTER OUTLINE

The following chapters outline my argument and provide a chronological and thematic discussion of the ways in which the process of remedicalization has taken place.

The process of remedicalization was in part driven by scientific and technological advances and developing disciplines. From the 1970s onwards, medicinal chemists, pharmacologists, sociologists and psychiatrists, neurologists, and anaesthetists all contributed to our understanding of cannabis and to its application as a medicine. This took place within the context of the rise of new specialist disciplines, such as clinical pharmacology, psychopharmacology, and phytopharmacy. Chapters 1 and 2 trace the changing understandings of cannabis.

Chapter 1 begins in the laboratory, with the emergence of interest in cannabis research just prior to the removal of cannabis tincture's PLR in 1973, whereby cannabis became illegal as a medicine. Awareness of cannabis had been raised through increased recreational use and the subsequent demand for drug control driving the need for a better understanding of cannabis. In turn, the scientific understanding of cannabis filtered through to discussions over cannabis's position within the control mechanisms. Through an analysis of archival material, I explore the work and influence of Sir W.D.M. Paton, a British pharmacologist who carried out important early work on cannabis, improving understanding of the pharmacological properties of the drug.

Scientific advances, such as in medicinal chemistry with the discovery of THC, opened up new avenues for research. Drug control laws posed a problem for researchers because they impacted on the availability and quality of raw material for research, but when these hindrances were partially overcome in the 1970s, laboratory research on the chemistry and pharmacology of cannabis began to progress and expand the fundamental understanding of the drug. This research placed emphasis on the harms associated with cannabis, especially potentially detrimental long-term effects. Therapeutic applications emerged, but for researchers like Paton, who placed emphasis on the precautionary principle, such applications were risky.

Chapter 2 takes up the story in the clinic, where there was renewed interest in cannabis's therapeutic properties within the context of the development of clinical pharmacology as a discipline. This chapter considers the role played by J.D.P. Graham, a clinical pharmacologist who began to write more positively about the drug and who was influential in expert discussions on cannabis in the 1970s. Driven by the need to find alternative effective treatments, clinicians then accepted cannabis as a therapeutic for the alleviation of the nausea associated with cancer chemotherapy; this contributed to the re-establishment of cannabis as a medicine in the United Kingdom through the limited approval of a single-chemical-entity drug. By 1982, however, failure to understand cannabis's mode of action, as well as changing public health priorities, drew scientists away from cannabis research.

The transfer of this new scientific knowledge to the policy environment through the developing mechanism of expert advice via expert committees is the subject of chapter 3. In the 1970s and 1980s committees were set up to give policy a stronger evidence base, especially in the illicit drugs field with the establishment of the ACMD. Through an examination of three distinct periods of the ACMD, the chapter considers shifting attitudes towards the control of cannabis in the policy environment and the interplay between science and policy, in particular the growing role of cannabis therapeutics within discussions, as well as the impact of the policy environment on the process of remedicalization. Although international and domestic drug control systems acted as a countervailing force against the medical use of cannabis, at the same time they provided the impetus for remedicalization. Treating cannabis as an illicit drug necessitated improving the knowledge base for control purposes, pulling scarce resources into the cannabis arena. As cannabis began to regain medical credibility, policymakers saw the advantage to be gained from recreating the dual role for cannabis, as it offered the opportunity to split medical from recreational use and, in the process, weaken demands for legalization. In the United Kingdom this was through a pharmaceutical provision.

Chapter 4 therefore explores how the pharmaceutical industry played a key role in the United Kingdom in facilitating an acceptable transition of cannabis as a therapeutic from self-help or kitchen physic to the clinic and then into the marketplace. The chapter charts the progression from the pharmaceutical industry's initial lack of interest in cannabis to a temporary interest that yielded the first licensed synthetic cannabis-based drugs, providing important materials for academic research and thus facilitating a breakthrough in the understanding of cannabis's mode of action. This breakthrough provided the foundation for a more sustained interest in cannabis therapeutics in the 1990s, and industry involvement then increased worldwide.

Chapter 4 centres on the story of a small UK biotechnology firm, GW Pharmaceuticals, and places it within the context of the rise of phytopharmacy. GW Pharmaceuticals exemplifies the interest in cannabis from the domestic pharmaceutical industry, and it drew inspiration from an interest in botanical substances, refocusing the spotlight on extracts of cannabis rather than single-chemical-entity substances. Industry production of CBMS appeared to offer a way of accepting cannabis's medical utility, at the same time as transferring ownership from 'illicit' drug users to the professional medical sphere by putting in place medical and regulatory structures around cannabis-based drugs. Within this, the form of cannabis that was utilized, developments in technology and delivery systems, and standardization were crucial. The ability to deliver cannabis via a new delivery system proved important. In the 1990s GW's new delivery system – an oral-mucosal spray – offered a number of advantages. It avoided smoked cannabis – a no-go for policymakers and the medical community – and it bypassed the problems associated with oral administration that had beset the single-chemical-entity drugs, instead providing patients with something more akin to the advantages of smoked cannabis.

Chapter 5 traces the role of lay advocacy in the remedicalization of cannabis in Western practices, particularly those in the United Kingdom, from the 1970s onwards. Activism began via drug liberalization demands, of which therapeutic cannabis was one aspect, and developed in the 1980s and early 1990s into specific campaigns for cannabis therapeutics in the United States: the concept of medical necessity developed in relation to glaucoma, cancer, and AIDS, for example. In the United Kingdom, MS patient associations, which campaigned for research into and access to cannabis in the 1990s, were influential in the scientific, clinical, industrial, and policy spheres. High-profile advocacy placed pressure on policymakers, and the outcome changed attitudes in government towards clinical trials and provided incentives for the pharmaceutical industry to become involved. Significant within this was the emphasis by MS campaigners on 'respectability' along with their ability to forge cross-class alliances. Following interviews from key insiders in the campaigns, this chapter argues that advocacy was crucial in focusing the direction of research and also in making research into extracts of cannabis imperative. Activism was important in forcing researchers, industry, and regulators to take account of the patient perspective, which is no small feat in medicine.

Cannabis therapeutics in the United Kingdom after the 1990s would not have advanced as it did without the legitimacy conferred on the concept by influential professional bodies such as the Royal Pharmaceutical Society (RPS), the BMA, and the House of Lords Science and Technology Committee. Chapter 6 continues the story of expert advice and the relationship between science and policy, but it also moves the story forward to consider the role of professional bodies and expert advice in the period 1997–2004. I trace the expert discussions through pivotal reports that emerged from the BMA and the House of Lords in the late 1990s, as well as discussions over the scheduling of cannabis in the MDA after the turn of the millennium. The chapter explores the impact of developments in the medical use of cannabis on the policy environment and also their impact on the debates about the process of remedicalization itself.

Evidence, clinical trials, and regulation are the subjects of chapter 7. In the 1980s, clinical trials of synthetic cannabinoids resulted in the licit licensed CBMs dronabinol (Marinol) and nabilone (Cesamet). These medicines largely focused on providing relief from the nausea experienced by chemotherapy patients. In the United

Kingdom further clinical trials on cannabis emerged after the convergence of interests post-1997, when the government agreed to permit the licensing of CBMs if they proved successful in clinical trials. The trials after 2000 – both industry trials and the proof-of-principle trials – brought extracts of cannabis rather than synthetic, single-entity cannabinoids into clinical trials for the first time. The trials, which struggled to show efficacy, nevertheless indicated limited adverse effects and some potential benefits. Significantly, though, they highlighted the methodological problems that clinical trials posed for cannabis and its derivatives: notably, the problems of studying a drug that was based on a readily available illicit substance, the perils of studying plants, and regulation.

The trials led to an acknowledgement of the limitation of available methods for measuring symptoms and problems such as chronic pain, and they also led to the development of improved patient-based outcome measures, which in turn, it was hoped, could lead to more successful outcomes for CBMs in future trials. The successful licensing of Sativex in Canada, and also the proof-of-principle trials in the United Kingdom, extended the application of cannabis beyond its anti-emetic properties to the treatment of MS and pain, and potentially towards neuro-protective aspects in the future. Clinical trials left various options open for licit CBMs, either through the development of existent synthetic products or through the emergent cannabis-based extracts such as Sativex; but trials did not yet open the door to patient access.

The book's final chapter brings together my key themes to look at the major developments in the last decade. Cannabis's continued borderline status created a backlash in policy circles, and within four years of being downgraded to class C it was regraded to class B in 2009, on the grounds of the availability of more potent strains and its threat to mental health. The mechanism of expert advice came in for criticism. With new pharmaceutical-grade cannabis-based drugs not made widely available, patients continued to pressure for access, forcing rapid changes in policy and questioning what constitutes 'evidence'.

In 2017 the UK MS Society changed its earlier position and called for herbal cannabis to be legalized for MS patients. In 2017–18 debate focused around cannabis for severe and rare forms of epilepsy in children, as seen in the high-profile cases of Alfie Dingley and Billy Caldwell, whose parents campaigned for access to cannabis oil, which they could obtain abroad but not at home. These medical imperatives quickly led to shifts in policy, resulting in cannabis-derived medicinal products being rescheduled from Schedule I to Schedule II at the end of 2018. This allowed the prescription of CBM in certain circumstances via doctors listed on the General Medical Council's special register. But because few of these products were either licensed by the Medicines and Healthcare products Regulatory Agency (MHRA) or approved by the National Institute for Health and Care Excellence (NICE), few have been prescribed.

Uncertainly around safety and efficacy have continued to pose a problem. In 2019 the UK Committee on Social Care argued that the research base remained limited because clinical trials were restricted under the previous scheduling and stressed that new trials were urgently needed. The committee called on the government 'to desist from confiscating prescribed medicinal cannabis provided overseas under specialist supervision'. In November 2019 NICE changed its guidelines to allow two CBMs to be used to treat two forms of epilepsy and MS, but not for other conditions such as chronic pain, and some patients' groups called it a missed opportunity. In response, Epidyolex, a cannabidiol-based (CBD-based) medicine, was fast-tracked to be made available in January 2020. For now, remedicalization remains an ongoing process with continuing issues around patient access.

METHODOLOGY

This book is heavily archival and interview-based. The National Archives at Kew in England provided a rich source of material, especially on the ACMD. Material held at the Wellcome Library provided a valuable collection of previously unstudied papers by researchers and organizations, such as those of Sir W.D.M. Paton, including personal correspondence, newspaper cuttings, and minutes of committees and expert groups on cannabis, as well as the archives for the MS Society from 1953 to 1977. The WHO Library and Archive in Geneva provided insight into international agency discussions.

Key interviewees proved helpful in providing additional information to that which could be located in libraries and archives, including personal papers, notes, correspondence, minutes, media cuttings, and funding applications. The archives of professional institutions, such as that of the RPS, yielded reports and minutes of the professional institutions that were involved in crucial events. Key reports of the organizations involved were analysed, including those from the House of Lords, the BMA, the WHO, the INCB, and the Department of Health. A timeline of major events was developed early on and the parliamentary record was reviewed, focusing on key events such as the reports of the ACMD. Media responses were surveyed, with a focus on two quality papers (*The Times* and *The Guardian*), two popular dailies (the *Daily Mirror* and the *Daily Mail*), and one Sunday paper (the *Independent on Sunday*).

Interviews with key interviewees included scientists, clinicians, policymakers, and activists, and these provided an enlightening source of material in addition to printed sources.[70,71] Interviews were supplemented by the organization of a witness seminar, a useful tool to draw together those involved in the field to discuss developments and to highlight tensions, debates, and networks.[72]

A WORD ON TERMINOLOGY

The terminology used to describe cannabis and its derivatives is complex. The words 'medicine' and 'drug' have often been used interchangeably, but this is not always appropriate. The term 'drug' has become increasingly linked to illicit recreational substances, whereas traditionally the term would have been applied to the active ingredient of a medicine. Terms such as 'pharmaceutics' and 'therapeutics' also confuse the issue.

In terms of cannabis specifically, there are different terms in common use for the plant: cannabis, marihuana, marijuana, ganja, as well as the more common parlance of pot, weed, grass, or skunk. These terms are generally used to refer to the dried flowers, stems, or leaves of female cannabis plants. I have used the UK version throughout, thus referring to 'cannabis' even when discussion of American developments refers to marijuana.

The term cannabis can also cover a number of different cannabis species, such as *Cannabis indica* and *Cannabis sativa*. Different versions have been more popular at different times and in different places, and each version has different components and effects. Hemp, for example, refers to the variant that does not contain a psychoactive element, and in Europe it was most widely used in rigging for ships' sails. Then there are the terms that refer to parts of cannabis in relation to their non-medical use, such as cannabis resin or hashish, a substance produced from the resin of the flowers that produces a more potent substance than the dried leaves.

Cannabis can contain more than sixty compounds termed cannabinoids (since 1999 the term phytocannabinoids has also been suggested). Examples include CBD, which accounts for up to 40 per cent of the plant's extract but which does not have psychoactive properties, and CBN, or delta-9-THC, which is the primary psychoactive element. Phytocannabinoids or phytomedicines are those extracted from a plant. Different variants and different growing conditions can lead to the production of different amounts of these constituents. Several medicines have been developed from cannabis. For the sake of simplicity I refer to CBMs, otherwise known as CBMPs, following the definition set out by the UK government in its 2018 Misuse of Drugs Regulations: '[A CBM is] a product that contains cannabis, cannabis resin, cannabinol or a cannabinol derivative (not being dronabinol or its stereoisomers); produced for medicinal use in humans and is a medicinal product, or a substance or preparation for use as an ingredient of, or in the production of an ingredient of, a medicinal product.'

The term CBMP can cover a variety of different products. The flowers, stems, or leaves of cannabis were originally used as a medicine, either smoked (often combined with tobacco) or taken as a tea. In this instance I have used the terms herbal, whole, or botanical cannabis. Common in the nineteenth century was the use of cannabis extract – that is, extracts of cannabis in alcohol prepared by percolation – or cannabis tincture, prepared by a dilution of cannabis extract.

From 1973 interest focused on the active psychoactive principle of cannabis, THC. This was followed by the development of synthetic versions of THC, usually administered in tablet form, e.g. nabilone (Cesamet), or a synthetic cannabinoid similar to THC called dronabinol (Marinol). Sativex is a cannabis-based medicine extract (CBME) that contains a mix of phytocannabinoids including CBD and CBN and is delivered in spray form. Epidyolex contains plant-based CBD.

'Cannabis preparation' refers to any cannabis medicine derived from cannabis that does not have marketing authorization as a medicinal project. This includes items such as tinctures or oils or raw cannabis, including the flowers. The term cannabis-based products for medical use in humans (CBPM) had emerged by 2020. As defined in Regulation 2(1) of the Misuse of Drugs Regulations 2001, a

CBPM is or contains cannabis, cannabis resin, cannabinol, or a cannabinol derivative; is produced for medicinal use in humans; and is regulated as a medicinal product, or an ingredient of a medicinal product. This splits down further as there are unlicensed CBPMs, which are products that have not been assessed by the MHRA. For example, Tilray's cannabidiol (CBD) oil. Licensed CBPMs are those that have been granted a marketing authorization but still fall under the definition of a CBPM. In contrast, licensed cannabis-based medicines (L-CBM) are products that have been granted marketing authorization by the medicines regulator (the MHRA or the EMA) and are scheduled under the MDR and are not classed as CBPMs. These include the drugs Epidyolex, nabilone, and Sativex. In the last few years, 'cannabis items' have appeared on the market. These are offered for sale on the basis that they are not psychoactive and might be referred to as 'cannabis light', e.g. CBD oil. These are often associated with health and well-being as opposed to medical purposes.

Remedicalization very much remains an ongoing process. In addition to being a story of a plant, an illicit drug, and a medicine, it is also the story of developing disciplines, national and commercial interests, patient perspectives, and 'evidence'. Emergent CBMs appeared to be able to exist within the drug control systems, and questions have shifted to the broader picture of the relative positions taken on the harm of both illicit and licit drugs and on the entire framework of control. Uncertainty has been crucial in the story of the process of remedicalization,[73] and where therapeutic cannabis will go from the point at which this study ends is unclear. This historical approach provides a window into an ongoing international process.

Understanding Cannabis: Pharmacology, Laboratory Research, and Drug Control, 1964–82

The early 1970s saw the development of parallel worlds around cannabis. On the one hand, international and national drug control policies were tightened, and cannabis was dropped as a medical product by 1973. Yet, on the other hand, as these moves took place, scientific interest in cannabis re-emerged. The search engine PubMed reveals that only 30 articles referred to cannabis during the 1950s, whereas 130 articles published between 1960 and 1970 did so. When cannabis was introduced to Britain as a medical product, its use was limited for several reasons: an undiscovered active principle, an inability to use it within new drug-delivery systems or to standardize the product, questionable efficacy, and fears over its side effects. By the time cannabis was removed as a medical product some of these problems had been solved and the door was opened to the reintroduction of CBMs.

This chapter focuses on early laboratory research and the role of one eminent British pharmacologist, Sir W.D.M. Paton, as a means of analysing the impact of changing scientific knowledge on the process of remedicalization. The chapter charts the re-emergence of interest in cannabis stimulated by breakthroughs in understanding its chemistry and pharmacology. It considers how the growth of recreational use led to the need for a greater scientific understanding of cannabis, in order to provide the evidence base to underpin drug control mechanisms. It highlights key debates around drug control and the transfer of knowledge between research in the laboratory and the development of drug control mechanisms. The chapter demonstrates how hindrances to research were partially overcome, enabling laboratory research on the chemistry and pharmacology of cannabis to be undertaken. It concludes by considering the impact of this pharmacological research and demonstrating how this early work in the laboratory laid the groundwork for moving from the laboratory to the clinic, allowing research on medical applications of cannabis to emerge.

THE DISCOVERY OF THE ACTIVE PRINCIPLE: OPENING THE DOOR TO CANNABIS RESEARCH

The recreational use of cannabis in the United Kingdom, a country where it had not previously been widely used, rapidly expanded in the 1960s and 1970s. This occurred in the context of a youth-driven cultural revolution, with shifts in cultural norms towards a more 'permissive' society. I focus on scientific developments here, but many authors have written on the growth of recreational cannabis use in both the United Kingdom and the United States, as well as on the development of cannabis cultures.[1] This increased recreational use brought cannabis to the fore of drug policy concerns and, in so doing, drove the development of scientific knowledge about the plant.

In the late 1950s the CND (the UN organization) had called for governments to encourage research into the active principles of cannabis, most notably in order to facilitate the accurate and speedy identification of dangerous parts of the plant, to combat illicit traffic.[2] The lack of an isolated, pure active principle had been a major hindrance to cannabis's use as a medicine, but this changed following a 1964 breakthrough in the work of the medicinal chemist Raphael Mechoulam and his group at the Hebrew University in Jerusalem, Israel.[3] Mechoulam discovered more about the plant's chemistry: he was interested in the chemistry and biological activity of natural products and synthetic drugs, having previously investigated several natural products including cannabinoids at the Weizmann Institute.

Mechoulam was surprised to find that, unlike the chemistries of morphine and cocaine, which were well known, the active compounds in cannabis had never been isolated in a pure form, nor were their structures really understood.[4] As he worked on its chemistry, Mechoulam achieved a major breakthrough: the isolation of

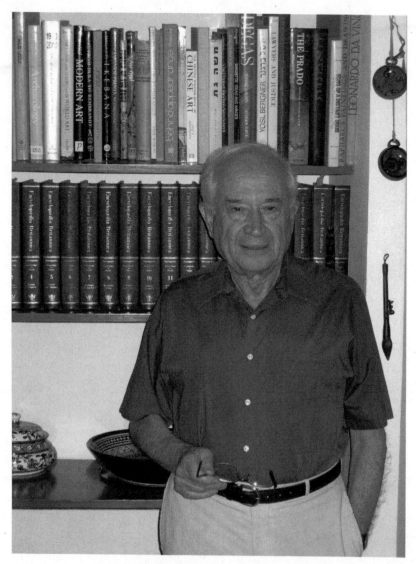

Figure 1.1   Professor Raphael Mechoulam.

the major psychoactive principle of cannabis, delta-9-THC.[5] This enabled him to elucidate its structure and stereochemistry.[6] He was
able to synthesize the active principle, and THC became available
in natural form via the plant and by way of synthesis. Researchers no longer had to rely on the plant material or on extracts of

cannabis with unknown constituents. THC could be produced from laboratory-made chemicals, which allowed the production of a standardized product, which was crucial for research and remedicalization. These two steps sparked interest in cannabis research and opened up funding possibilities. Mechoulam noted the change:

> When we started nobody was interested. We couldn't get
> a penny to do research on it ... The Americans told me
> that it's a South American problem, we are not interested.
> Then everyone was interested in it, and I was supported in
> my research for nearly forty years by the National Institutes
> of Health (NIH) in the US. They were interested in the
> chemistry of course ... we supplied them with materials
> in the beginning ... gave them the first ten grams and on
> this material quite a lot of work was done in the US in the
> 1960s and probably the 70s.[7]

NIDA, created in 1972 as part of the National Institutes of Health (NIH), began supplying cannabis to scientists; it also provided 85 per cent of the world's research dollars for cannabis research.[8] Besides Mechoulam's discovery, little else was known about cannabis and the effect of cannabinoids such as THC: research was thus necessary in the areas of pharmacology and epidemiology. Furthermore, these new cannabinoids posed problems for drug control policies, as they were outside the control mechanisms, having been discovered after the 1961 Single Convention on Narcotic Drugs.

DRUG CONTROL, THE MEDICAL RESEARCH COUNCIL, AND SIR W.D.M. PATON, 1968–70

Paton was one of the first researchers in the United Kingdom to expand pharmacological knowledge around cannabis and cannabinoids, publishing significant texts throughout the 1970s. Although the 'great man' method of biography and approach to history has its criticisms, a study of Paton's work on the pharmacology of cannabis provides a lens through which we can understand pivotal issues around cannabis research. Paton, who kept prolific notes of his work, is important not only for his contribution to the expansion of scientific knowledge around cannabis, but also for his endeavours to transfer that knowledge to drug policy.

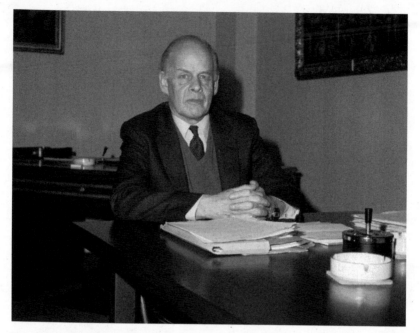

Figure 1.2   Sir William Drummond Macdonald Paton.

William Drummond Macdonald Paton was born in Hendon in the United Kingdom in 1917, and he trained in medicine at Oxford University. After suffering bouts of pneumonia, he moved away from the clinical field into pharmacology. He became a member of staff at the National Institute for Medical Research between 1944 and 1952 and went on to become Reader in pharmacology at University College Hospital, London, between 1952 and 1954. He then became Professor of Pharmacology at the Royal College of Surgeons, London, staying there until 1959, and he was made a Fellow of the Royal Society in 1956.

Paton's early work in experimental pharmacology – such as that on methonium compounds with the pharmacologist Eleanor Zaimis – and his collaboration with anaesthetist Geoffrey Organe led to important discoveries in the drug treatment of hypertension and the pharmacology of smooth muscle relaxants.[9] He become Professor of Pharmacology at the University of Oxford and a Fellow of Balliol College, Oxford between 1959 and 1984.

His other previous work had focused on decompression sickness, on which he acted as a consultant to the Royal Navy. As part of this work he was interested in anaesthetic mechanisms, and, during his time at Oxford, Paton was able to overcome some of the problems of deep-sea diving through his research on the physiological properties of gases at high pressure, which led to the development of Trimix (oxygen, helium, and nitrogen) for divers. This interest in anaesthetic mechanisms later informed his research on cannabis. Much of his work at Oxford focused on drug dependence and, in particular, the pharmacology of cannabis. He was sought after by the government and by professional bodies, and he sat on more than seventy committees. He was knighted in 1979.

A significant factor determining the direction of his research on cannabis was that Paton came to the study of its pharmacology via an interest in drug dependence.[10] At the time, concepts around drug use were fluid. Perceptions had shifted from the concept of 'habit-forming' drugs to 'addiction' in the post-war period, and in 1964 the World Health Organization (WHO) recommended the use of the term 'drug dependence' rather than addiction.[11] The term 'addiction' was associated with the idea of withdrawal symptoms and a developing tolerance to a drug, as seen with the use of opiates. The concept of 'dependence' merged the concepts of habituation and addiction. It was viewed as a broader model, referring to drugs that maintained some hold on the user through either physical or psychic characteristics. Prior to the 1960s, drug dependence had been considered in relation to alcohol and tobacco, but in the 1960s non-medical use of illicit drugs expanded considerably in the United Kingdom, becoming a topic of major concern.[12]

Paton considered cannabis to be a drug of dependence of the 'psychic type'. He recognized that critics might view this as an overreaction: 'I am sure it is true that the dependence is not normally strong and some might think I make too much of it.' However, he viewed it as one of the most dangerous of the dependence-producing drugs because he thought it was innocuous enough to enter general circulation, unlike drugs such as lysergic acid diethylamide (LSD), which had side effects that he thought would deter most potential users.[13] When Paton wrote on drug dependence in 1968, he emphasized that cannabis was not understood well enough to inform policy. For this reason, in his advisory capacity he consistently pressured for the maintenance of the status quo in the legal situation around cannabis.[14] Much of Paton's early work had been funded by his department in Oxford, but in 1969 Paton applied for and received funding for two years from the Medical Research Council (MRC) to investigate the actions and toxicity of cannabis.[15] But why were Paton and the MRC interested in cannabis research and its funding?

The incentive to study the pharmacology of cannabis was driven by drug control imperatives, not medical need: medical use and research were constrained by control policies introduced to restrain recreational drug use. In the 1960s and 1970s the policy environment around drugs, and especially cannabis, was in flux. The UN Single Convention on Narcotic Drugs of 1961 simplified earlier control regimes and expanded controls to cover plants from which 'narcotic' drugs were produced.[16] It was a continuation and consolidation of the 'dominant supply control mentality'.[17] It introduced a scheduling system with substances placed within four Schedules, of which Schedule I and Schedule IV were the most restrictive (for more information, see the lists of Schedules in the introduction). The convention meant that controlled drugs could only be used for medical and scientific purposes, though countries in which a drug had 'traditional uses' were exempted for twenty-five years.

Medical use was an important delineator for the placement of a drug within the control system. Analysis of documents and reports from the international agencies shows how, in drafting the new drug legislation, policy impacted the medical use of cannabis for the first time. The documents indicate that the WHO – the UN health body responsible for advising the CND and the central policymaking body of the UN for drug-related matters – was hostile to medical cannabis.

This was significant because the WHO was responsible for making recommendations to the CND on the level of international control that should be applied to 'dependence-producing drugs'. In 1952 a WHO expert committee informed the CND that there was no justification for the medical use of cannabis.[18] This decision was important, as it was the first time cannabis had been officially declared to have no medical role; previously, it had simply fallen out of widespread medical use. When, in 1953, the CND asked the WHO to consider the mental and physical effects of cannabis, the WHO condemned the drug unequivocally, and the UN Economic and Social Council urged governments to discontinue its use as a medicine. This advice paved the way for the CND to severely curtail the use of cannabis, and by 1957 the CND had requested the prohibition of all but traditional medical uses.[19] This was critical because it meant that

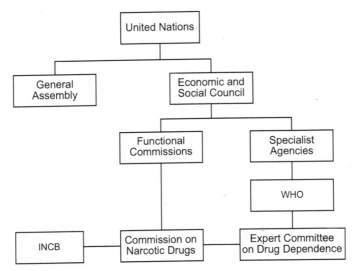

Figure 1.3   United Nations system and drug control organs and their secretariat.

cannabis was differentiated from heroin and its medical derivative diamorphine, which were seen as having some medical properties despite attempts to ban their medical use.[20]

Yet, while these international control mechanisms around cannabis were being tightened, research on cannabis continued. Research in Eastern Europe indicated some potential medical uses, for instance as an antibiotic.[21] Such research filtered through to the CND, which expressed concern that the draft of a planned new drug control convention might limit medical uses, and as a result it requested that the WHO re-examine cannabis's medical utility.[22] But when the WHO reviewed the antibiotic properties of cannabis it found no reason to backtrack on its original assessment.[23] Cannabis and cannabis tincture, extracts, and resin were placed in Schedule I of the Single Convention. This placed it in the same category as morphine, and it permitted medical use. But unlike morphine, cannabis and cannabis resin were also placed in Schedule IV, on the grounds that medical use was 'obsolete' and that its recreational use was allegedly widespread. For Schedule IV the convention required parties to prohibit the cultivation, production, manufacture, export and import, trade, possession, and use of the drug (except for research purposes).[24] Penalties for misuse were left under the control of domestic laws. This led to different interpretations of the convention in different countries. Cannabis was left in a vulnerable position by the WHO's decision to discount its medical utility.

Governments were required to implement punitive legislation for drug misuse. This led to the establishment of the 1964 UK Drugs (Prevention of Misuse) Act and the 1965 DDA, which consolidated previous legislation. The 1964 Act replicated the Schedules of the UN convention. It regulated the import, export, manufacture, sale, and possession of cannabis, morphine, and opium, and it extended controls to cannabis and coca leaves; by 1967 subsequent legislation had also introduced police powers to stop and search drug suspects. These policy measures created incentives to better understand the drugs under control and the impact of this control. Cannabis in particular posed a problem for legislators, especially as there were large numbers of young people in the 1960s receiving criminal convictions for possession.[25] In the United Kingdom, where recreational use had been limited prior to the 1960s, its use increased despite tighter cannabis regulation, and cannabis control became a priority for drug regulators and expert committees.

One expert committee drew attention to the problems that cannabis posed to the drug control systems. In 1967 the Sub-committee on Hallucinogens of the Advisory Committee on Drug Dependence (ACDD), chaired by Baroness Wootton, a leading British sociologist and criminologist, had delved into the available evidence on the pharmacological, clinical, pathological, social, and legal aspects of these drugs and produced a report focused on cannabis. The Wootton Report concurred that in terms of physical harm cannabis was a dangerous drug, but it questioned the harm of cannabis in comparison with other drugs, both licit and illicit: 'In terms of physical harmfulness, cannabis is very much less dangerous than the opiates, amphetamines and barbiturates, and also less dangerous than alcohol.'[26]

Moderate use of cannabis was not seen as especially harmful. Flexibility in the drug control system was deemed necessary: 'We do not wish to make any formal or absolute statement on a comparison of cannabis and the other drugs in common social use. All we would wish to say is that the gradations of danger between consuming tea and coffee at one end of the scale and injecting heroin intravenously at the other, may not be permanently those which we now ascribe to particular drugs.'[27] The Wootton Report concluded that there was no convincing evidence for the 'gateway theory'. The gateway theory implied that there was a sequence of drug use, where cannabis would lead to the use of other 'harder' hallucinogenic drugs; the theory was often used in policy discussions to justify strict controls and penalties on cannabis use.[28] The report recommended that in the interests of public health it was necessary to maintain restrictions on the availability of cannabis, but it argued that the law should be recast to give more flexible control over individual drugs. It called for new legislation to deal with cannabis separately, isolating it from drugs such as the opiates. It questioned the perceived dangers of cannabis use and the penalties applied to cannabis under the criminal justice system.[29]

The sub-committee saw no problem with cannabis as a prescribed legal medicine: 'We see no objection to this and believe that any new legislation should be such as to permit its continuance.'[30] The new synthetic versions of cannabinoids such as THC had opened up a new dimension to the debate, and these versions were seen as worthy of investigation.[31] The sub-committee's recommendation for a reconsideration of drug policy and its call for an improved scientific base that reduced research constraints stimulated research into cannabis, which indirectly stimulated research into cannabis therapeutics.[32]

The government quickly rejected the Wootton Report. It accepted some elements: the problems caused by the police powers of stop and search were viewed with concern, for example, and discussion of this aspect was passed back to the ACDD.[33] The extent to which the government could change legislation was limited since it was a signatory to the UN Single Convention on Narcotic Drugs of 1961. Although James Callaghan, the Home Secretary, rejected calls for decriminalization, he did accept the need for cannabis research, and he called for the subsequent involvement of the MRC: 'I fully accept that more comprehensive and flexible powers of control are needed to check drug abuse … We also accept that there is a need for wider research and we are bringing this to the notice of the Research Council.'[34] Cannabis remained a controlled drug, but the penalties associated with its use came under scrutiny in the following years and the MRC became deeply involved in cannabis research.[35]

The MRC had its origins at the beginning of the twentieth century in the search for solutions to the threat of tuberculosis (TB). It had come into independent being after World War I with a remit to fund research into public health threats. As the public health focus shifted from infectious disease to lifestyle disease, the MRC's attention fell on the problems associated with growing recreational drug use. But its interest in psychopharmacology, a discipline that was developing in the 1970s, arose from a long-standing interest in basic laboratory work.[36] The MRC had outlined its policy in 1969, stating that it was 'most anxious to foster a comprehensive research programme on the various aspects of drug dependence'.[37] The MRC had previously called a conference in 1967 to determine avenues for future research, and it subsequently established three working parties to consider the research needs around drug dependence: the Working Party on Biochemical and Pharmacological Aspects of Drug Dependence, the Working Party on the Evaluation of Different Methods of Treatment of Drug Dependence, and the Working Party on the Epidemiology of Drug Dependence.[38]

The Working Party on Biochemical and Pharmacological Aspects of Drug Dependence, which met for the first time in 1969, was chaired by Sir W.D.M. Paton. It was composed of leading academics in their field, including Dr Marley from the Institute of Psychiatry, Maudsley Hospital; Professor A.H. Beckett from the Department of Pharmacy, Chelsea College; Dr Graham from the Department of Pharmacology, the Welsh National School for Medicine; Professor Gray, a consultant chemical pathologist from King's College London; Dr Johnston, a Ministry of Health observer; an observer from the Scottish Home and Health Department; and G.S. Geoffrey, a Home Office observer. Its terms of reference were to focus on the need for research into the biochemistry and pharmacology of drug dependence; to work out which areas were of priority; and to recommend what research should be encouraged.[39]

During its operation it was asked to comment on some of the recommendations made by the Wootton Report. By the late 1970s there was pressure for additional drugs legislation, and a draft proposal was produced. Existing legislation was seen as 'uncoordinated, inflexible, and inadequate.' New legislation sought to control the availability of any drug, the misuse of which both caused ill effects to the individual and constituted a public health and social problem. Some drugs were to be subject to controls based on their comparative harms and circumstance of misuse. It was expected that most of these would be pharmaceutical products with accepted medical or scientific uses, but legislation would also include those that might be used for non-therapeutic use.[40] Importantly, it was not expected that the controls would apply to licit, widely used drugs such as alcohol, tobacco, tea, or coffee, as Paton later queried.

The Home Office prepared a confidential report and asked the MRC for comments, and the MRC in turn passed the report on to the chairmen of the sub-committees.[41] Paton's response to the report, which was subsequently forwarded to Mr Turner at the Home Office, provides an interesting insight into the debates over the drug control framework.[42] Paton drew the distinction between what might be desirable and what might be practical: 'Fundamentally I think the approach is sound and as I understand it would allow much more flexibility in dealing with a situation liable to change rather rapidly ... I find myself in a dilemma. On the one hand, I think it is probably sensible to be able to separate the more harmful from the less harmful drugs. On the other hand, I am not sure that it is easy to do operationally.'[43] Paton raised prescient points in terms of the assessment of harm and the separation of drugs. He deemed the flexibility of the system to be important, citing the changing knowledge over amphetamines. He queried where the lines could and should be drawn between derivatives. Where, for example, would the line be drawn in the sequence of opiate-based drugs? Cannabis, Paton expected, would be placed in the least harmful category, although he noted that potential developments around synthetic cannabinoid administration might change this situation: 'Finally I am sure that cannabis and derivatives would be placed in the less harmful category but of course this is only just starting and I have little doubt that synthetic cannabinoids for intravenous administration will in due course appear and since I doubt if these could be regarded as less harmful than say a casual oral dose of pentazocide one might have got things the wrong way round.'[44] Flexibility of movement within the drug control mechanism would be of greater importance in later decades as scientific understanding expanded and the social use of drugs changed.

In looking for a solution to drug control, Paton queried if drug-delivery methods, rather than the drug itself, were the more pressing and controllable point: 'Accordingly I wonder whether it is possible to incorporate controls over more or less harmful methods of use.'[45] Later on, drug-delivery systems would become critical, providing a method by which medical cannabis could be differentiated from recreational use.

The Working Party on Biochemical and Pharmacological Drug Dependence looked at a variety of drugs and reported to the MRC in 1970. It became clear that cannabis was the least studied and understood drug of dependence, and it was this that triggered further calls for research into cannabis.[46] One area of particular concern was the lack of reliable tests for cannabis in the blood.[47] This aspect was deemed essential in the light of penalties imposed by the DDAS and the Drugs (Prevention of Misuse) Act.

The Working Party on the Epidemiology of Drug Dependence, was chaired by Professor M. Roth from the Department of Psychological Medicine, Newcastle University, and it considered the need for research on the epidemiology of drug dependence and made recommendations to the MRC on specific research projects that should be encouraged.[48] It concluded that there was insufficient research directed towards the problem of how and where drugs became available to the addict,[49] and that a focus on special groups such as adolescents in borstal[50] and young people at universities was desirable.[51]

The original working parties were disbanded and replaced by a new working party, chaired by Dr Owen, to facilitate action based on their recommendations. The interest in the biological aspects of drug dependence in relation to substances such as cannabis, nicotine, and alcohol remained important, and it was deemed to warrant the establishment of a separate working party that became the Working Party on the Biological Aspects of Drug Dependence. Established in 1971 and chaired by Paton, it considered the pharmacological issues that earlier working groups had not covered.[52] It was to look into the state of knowledge on the biochemistry and the pharmacology of dependence. It was also established to identify suitable teams already working or who might work in the area, and therefore to identify problems on which the MRC should contract research.[53] The working party pushed for further research, most notably to ascertain the fate of cannabis in the human body, and to develop reliable biochemical tests to assist with criminal prosecutions.

The MRC was to be critical in funding the clinical trials into therapeutic cannabis in later decades, but its interest began by funding research that improved the fundamental understanding of cannabis.[54] This necessitated pharmacological research. Pharmacology – the study of the effects of a drug on the body and the means by which it exerts its influence – had become the cornerstone of drug development. The British Pharmacological Society had been established in 1931, and psychopharmacology – a branch of pharmacology – had been developing since the 1950s. The discipline of pharmacology expanded in the 1960s, and psychopharmacology became of greater significance in the 1970s. Berridge showed that psychopharmacology, which focuses on psychoactive substances and their chemical interaction in the brain, became important to public health and led to the reintroduction of the role of 'laboratory medicine'.[55]

Paton was a firm believer that pharmacology was an intrinsic route to understanding psychoactive drugs.[56] When the Wootton Report was released in 1968, suggesting that cannabis should not be included in the DDA, Paton was against these conclusions on the grounds that there was little hard scientific evidence on which to make such a decision. Edward Gill, a colleague of Paton's, remembered that it was Lady Wootton's retort to Paton ('If there isn't that much pharmacology isn't it about time you did some?') that triggered the subsequent work done in the department of pharmacology at Oxford.[57] Paton and his team, funded by the MRC, would go on to carry out laboratory work there, answering vital previously unanswered pharmacological questions on cannabis.

OVERCOMING PROBLEMS OF SUPPLY FOR LABORATORY-BASED CANNABIS RESEARCH, 1969–73

Paton's pharmacological research required supplies of cannabis, but this was becoming increasingly complex. Controlled drugs could be made available as medicines, but the 1960s saw fears raised around the safety of chemicals such as DDT as well as licit medicinal drugs. Rachel Carson's *Silent Spring*, published in 1962, had awoken people to the impact of using dichloro-diphenyl-trichloroethane (DDT).[58] The thalidomide disaster in the same year revealed how medicines previously thought safe could pose an appalling threat to patients, and this shook people's confidence in drug therapy and existing regulation. The UK government determined to exert greater control over the provision of medicine, introducing the Medicines Act of 1968 to take account of the more potent medicines developed during the therapeutic revolution of the 1950s and 1960s. This Act gave the government the power to license pharmaceutical companies, products, and clinical trials.

The importance of the development of safety controls around medicines has been widely discussed by historians, and they certainly proved important in the process of remedicalization.[59] Under the new 1968 licensing system, medicines were given PLRs, which allowed drugs to be prescribed. PLRs were granted automatically to products already on the market when the Act came into force. Controlled drugs with medicinal value came under the control of the Medicines Act 1968 as well. Cannabis tincture automatically received a PLR, leaving it under the auspices of controlled drugs and medicines, and as such it was available to researchers. Gill recalled: 'There was a firm called Ransom ... that had the country's entire stock of tincture of cannabis. So, my job ... was simply to isolate a sample of pure THC.'[60]

But to isolate THC from the tincture was a time-consuming process. The 1970 annual report of the MRC discussed the problem: 'The extraction of significant quantities of pure derivatives from crude cannabis is a laborious undertaking and although it can be carried out in any good laboratory it is wasteful of time and manpower.'[61] The synthesis of THC had partially solved the problem by providing a standardized, industrial product, but supplies of THC were difficult to obtain.[62] Paton was mystified by Mechoulam's ability to source THC, and he wrote in 1969: 'I was fascinated by your remark about the relative availability of delta-9-THC ... when I looked into it a year ago there seemed to be none available and a notable silence on the topic, it shows again how one must know where to go!'[63] THC was not included in the 1961 UN Single Convention on Narcotic Drugs, and a Home Office licence was not required for its import, but it remained difficult to source.[64] The inclusion of cannabis in the 1961 Single Convention, however, had made the situation complicated. Mechoulam, for example, wished to send Paton some extracts, but Paton had to organize licences for the material to be shipped.[65] The alternative was to circumvent the bureaucracy and risk prosecution in order to maintain an informal supply between researchers.

Problems intensified with the introduction of the 1971 Convention on Psychotropic Substances. This convention brought in more comprehensive drugs regulation that amended the 1961 convention. The 1961 convention had generally been seen as a compromise and was subsequently superseded by drug developments, such as the introduction of pyschotropics, e.g. barbiturates, which often rapidly entered the medical sphere.[66] The 1971 convention retained the idea of Schedules but altered their significance. Schedule I took the place of Schedule IV as the most stringent one, including substances 'whose liability to abuse constitutes an especially serious risk to public health and which have very limited if any therapeutic usefulness'. Parties in the 1971 convention were required to provide punishable offences in domestic legislation. At the same time, the convention also reflected a greater focus on studying the nature of addiction and treatment. Thus, cannabis-based drugs including phytotetrahydrocannabinol appeared in Schedule I, and parties were therefore obliged to ban them 'except for scientific and very limited medical purposes by duly authorized persons'. Schedule I products were not acknowledged as having medical value.

How this worked in practice could vary between signatories. The United States had already placed cannabis in the most restrictive category: Schedule I of their domestic Controlled Substances Act of 1970, which included drugs deemed to be dangerous and without recognized medical use. The Netherlands, Canada, and some Australian states, on the other hand, took a more liberal approach. Britain introduced the 1971 MDA, which became the cornerstone of UK drug policy. It focused on the supply and possession of 'dangerous or otherwise harmful drugs', which became known as 'controlled drugs'. Schedule I of this Act introduced the ACMD, and Schedule II of this Act listed the controlled drugs.

The MDA, which came into force in 1973, was complex because it had to create a balance between permitting the 'correct use' of medically or scientifically useful controlled drugs and preventing their misuse. Under Schedule II of the Act, controlled drugs were classified into three classes, A, B, and C, with each classification determined by the severity of penalties that could be imposed. Drugs derived from cannabis, including cannabinoids such as cannabinol (CBN) or THC, were placed in the most restrictive class A, while herbal cannabis and cannabis resin were initially listed as class B, meaning that they could be used under licence from the Home Office for research purposes. To avoid having to amend the MDA there was provision for subordinate legislation to allow for amendments through its regulations. For example, regulations permitted exemptions for legitimate activities such as medical use.

Cannabis, certain psychoactive cannabinoids, and derivatives were not deemed to have medical use and were therefore not exempted under the regulations; they were thus placed in the most restrictive

classes, A and B, requiring a licence from the Home Office for research purposes. In contrast, substances such as morphine could be
exempt under the regulations and did not require a licence from
the Home Office for clinical trials. So, if a cannabis-based drug,
e.g. CBN, was to be made a commercially available licensed product, the drug needed to be transferred to a less restrictive class.
With no acknowledged medical use, cannabis lost its PLR and could
no longer be prescribed by doctors or dispensed by pharmacists,
though it could be used for research purposes with a Home Office
licence. This move meant that by 1973 cannabis came under the
sole control of illicit drug regulation. This proved problematic for
research but conversely also drew interest in the subject for drug
control imperatives.

As an illicit drug, supply of the raw material proved awkward for
researchers. Limited research–industry links created problems for
the supply chain, and MRC-funded projects ground to a halt due to
insufficient research materials. A domestic source of cannabis or
synthesized THC would have simplified the problem, but when the
MRC attempted to encourage a commercial firm to supply cannabis
under contract there was little optimism.[67] The supplies required
were small scale, so likely suppliers such as Miles Laboratories refused to become involved.[68]

The next option was to turn to an overseas source. The NIMH in
the United States had begun to fund research projects into cannabis, initially on the assumption that it would provide an evidence
base for the harms of cannabis use and would thus underpin control
policies. The NIMH was prepared to supply material free of charge,
but UK researchers perceived this as a problem as it left them reli-
ant on agreements with a foreign authority, one with its own policy
and research agenda. Furthermore, the US supply of cannabis was
rich in THC but lacked CBD, another important component of cannabis. Paton was deeply unconvinced about this supply chain and
complained to the MRC about reliance on the NIMH in 1971.[69] In
one letter he wrote: 'I do not care for leaving the decision whether
a project is worthy, not to the MRC but to NIMH ... I do not consider
consulting Dr Collier as adequately exploring the possibilities in industry ... If it becomes established that the MRC will not make its own
arrangements for supply then there is another possibility, that they
negotiate an agreement with NIMH whereby the latter makes available to the MRC a quantity for distribution at the MRC's discretion.'[70]

Hopes were briefly raised when it appeared that Imperial Chemical Industries (ICI) might be interested, particularly since its research director, D.G. Davey, had been co-opted on to the MRC. But this came to nothing as ICI found that the complexity of the operation did not justify the investment.[71] Expense and expertise waylaid other industrial alternatives. Davey suggested Koch-Light Laboratories, a maker of industrial fine chemicals in Suffolk. Paton rejected this idea on the grounds of expense, time constraints, and their lack of expertise.[72]

The inability to procure a domestic supply left three potential sources: Dr Olav Brænden, chief of the scientific and technical section of the Division of Narcotic Drugs at the UN; Dr Monique Braude, acting chief of the biomedical section of the NIMH; or Makor Chemicals, an Israeli producer. None of these sources appeared to be ideal: the UN source seemed to fall by the wayside; the NIMH source was advantageous in terms of costs but problematic in that there were conditions attached to the supply; and the Israeli source involved a commercial transaction.[73] As time went on, the cost and practicalities outweighed the concerns of obtaining supplies from the NIMH. Paton eventually resigned himself to a US supply though he remained dissatisfied, and he wrote to the MRC of his desire to source material from Europe: 'I have reservations about the work becoming wholly centred in the USA and wish there was an adequate source of supply in Europe. But the fact is the NIMH is willing to give it away.'[74]

The MRC had secured supplies from the NIMH by 1972 and began to act as the central liaison and distribution point.[75] Problems arose over how to obtain the necessary import licences from the Home Office. Additionally, the solution ignored non-MRC-funded researchers.[76] Although MRC researchers received the supply, there remained some dissatisfaction; for example, researchers were irritated that they could not supply other colleagues directly. The NIMH system was viewed merely as an interim solution. When the MRC wrote to researchers in 1973 to ask if they required additional material, researchers feared that the MRC wished to divest itself of this distributive role. Gill expressed his frustration with the system to the MRC:

> Research groups ... are inhibited by the difficulties in obtaining small quantities of pure materials ... Research groups could approach the NIMH directly but if a body with the authority and administrative resources of the

MRC find it tiresome to complete the port formalities
then the burden on individual departments is even
more severe. The Misuse of Drugs Act makes it illegal to
provide ... samples unless one goes to the considerable
trouble of obtaining a Home Office licence ... It would
... appear that the MRC is contemplating abandoning its
role as an intermediary ... If that is the case it is a most
unfortunate decision.[77]

The MRC agreed to maintain its role acting as a clearing house for
all UK requests. This early period opened the door to cannabis research, providing both incentives to study cannabis and systems for
doing so. But it revealed the serious consequences of a lack of domestic industry interest, and it limited research–industry relationships – a
gap that stakeholders were keen to fill in later decades; the emergence of UK industry interest in the 1990s is discussed in chapter 4.

The banning of cannabis tincture also impacted the direction
of research, as Roger Pertwee, a pharmacologist and colleague of
Paton's in the early 1970s, recalled: 'In the early 1970s tincture of
cannabis was banned. It was no longer a medicine. It had ceased.
And the main interest then for research was why is cannabis bad for
you? Why is it taken recreationally?'[78]

Research by psychologists expanded, with researchers such as
Adele Kosviner at the Addiction Research Unit, also funded by the
MRC, focusing on the prevalence and impact of cannabis use among
university students.[79] Nevertheless, the emphasis remained on establishing the pharmacology of cannabis.

EXPERIMENTAL PHARMACOLOGY AND
THE PROBLEMS OF CANNABIS USE

Basic pharmacological questions over cannabis remained unanswered in the early 1970s: What was its pharmacology? What kind
of impact did the structure of cannabis have? Was THC the main
psychoactive ingredient? What were the physiological effects of
cannabis and cannabinoids like THC? Paton argued that the role
of the pharmacologist in understanding psychoactive drugs was to
provide an overall description of a drug's actions to 'act as insur-
ance against adverse reactions in human practice'.[80] Throughout
the 1970s Paton and the group at Oxford started to answer some of

these questions by introducing *in vitro* studies of cannabis. *In vitro* studies provided a controlled environment for studying the effects of cannabis. Roger Pertwee described the initial focus of research as follows: 'Early pharmacology was descriptive because so little was known and you could go in any direction you liked and there would be new stuff to learn about what THC and cannabis were doing. A lot of interest was in confirming that THC was the main psychoactive constituent of cannabis by comparing the two pharmacologically.'[81]

Research sought to establish the effects of cannabis and individual cannabinoids on biological systems, especially cannabis's ability to cause dependence, and to compare cannabis with other drugs.[82] Paton and his group published preliminary results of their research in *Nature* in 1970, in which they confirmed that THC was the main psychoactive constituent of cannabis and that they found six other pharmacological effective components of cannabis.[83] They discovered that the effects of cannabis included lowered body temperature, catalepsy, analgesia, and, when combined with barbiturates, the extension of sleep. In the early 1970s cannabis's interaction with other drugs had become an important area of research. Paton and Pertwee continued to look at the effects of cannabis constituents on pentobarbitone sleeping time and phenazone metabolism. Building on pharmacological studies into cannabis's structure–activity relationship by Professor Sigmund Loewe in the 1940s and 1950s, they investigated the effect of cannabis on sleep induced by certain barbiturates.[84] They researched the mechanism of action of this effect in mice and then sought the constituents of cannabis responsible. Detailed results of the research were published in 1972. They found that cannabis extract prolonged sleep time and that the effect was dose related. They concluded that cannabis extract inhibited the microsomal activity of the mouse liver through the CBD content. It was also thought probable that human cannabis consumption could lead to interactions with other drugs, not merely barbiturates.

The group also developed new technology for studying cannabis. Pertwee had become interested in inert gas narcosis after doing a diving course with the military while at university. He went on to do his PhD under Paton on gas narcosis caused by diving and undertook post-doctorate work on cannabis, as it appeared to act similarly to anaesthetics.[85]

Pertwee developed a new quantitative method to assay cannabis biologically: a bioassay for cannabis. Bioassays measure the pharmacological activity of substances and are a prerequisite for establishing modes of action, a facet of cannabis that was not understood.[86] This bioassay tested the cataleptic effect of cannabis by measuring the percentage of time a mouse spent completely immobile on a horizontal wire ring. Pertwee established that responses were dose related, and he concluded that THC was largely responsible and that CBD had no effect. His test was demonstrated at a meeting of the British Pharmacological Society and was published in 1972.[87] The test, along with three others, was to form part of the Tetrad Tests, which became a mainstay of experiments on animals.

This was significant because bioassays tended to open up new research avenues, as had occurred in the tobacco and nicotine field.[88] In the early 1970s these new avenues tended to focus on the harmful effects of cannabis. Gill has described the legislative imperative and the funding focus on establishing harms: 'I think the main thrust of the work that was being done then was trying to establish there was a clear-cut case for decriminalizing cannabis. It is clearly difficult to prove a negative, i.e. to demonstrate that THC was not harmful, and one rather got the feeling that a lot of the work that was being financed was really to establish whether you could clearly demonstrate a harmful effect. If that was the case then that would really take care of the legislative problem ... The stuff was dangerous so it ought to be controlled.[89]

Research highlighted cannabis's potential problems and provided a degree of evidence to underpin the fears that had been raised in the nineteenth century. Although cannabis was not known to cause death, there were nevertheless concerns over its physical effects. Paton raised fears over toxicity in a 1972 research report for the MRC. He found that THC was the most toxic constituent of cannabis but that other cannabinoids, such as CBD, were also active and had observable effects. Animal experiments showed that the administration of cannabis caused weight loss, to which some animals adapted while others died. Paton noted the development of tolerance and the existence of withdrawal symptoms at high dosages in animals, and though they were not to the same degree as with barbiturates, he felt that this could still be sufficient to predispose continued use. This was significant because tolerance and withdrawal symptoms were considered diagnostic criteria for substance dependence. Paton's work raised fears that toxicity was likely to be cumulative, a result of the drug's fat-soluble (lipophilic) properties.

This was seen as having serious implications for cannabis use, especially over the long term.[90] For Paton, research that appeared to show cumulative and teratogenic effects in animals meant that the use of cannabis in humans was not acceptable until there was 'unequivocal evidence' that humans were not susceptible to the effects seen in animal research.[91]

Paton worked hard to publicize the results of his research and to carry his concerns to a wide audience. 'Cannabis and Its Problems', presented at the Royal Society of Medicine and published in the *Proceedings of the Royal Society of Medicine* in 1973, reviewed existing literature on the adverse effects of cannabis. Areas of concern included teratogenicity, carcinogenicity, and the impact on mental health.[92] He expanded on the behavioural effects on neurophysiology, putting these varied effects down to the 'disinhibiting action', which affected concentration and memory. In an analysis of the psychopathological problems, his paper raised the issue of 'cannabis psychosis', and he argued that, though the literature on this was rarely cited in contemporary debates around cannabis, it should be taken into account. However, he did draw distinctions between 'effects due simply to cannabis ... and exacerbation of a personality disorder, precipitation of psychosis and the exacerbation of pre-existing psychosis'.[93]

A key concern for Paton was the drug's effect on young people: the potentially cumulative effect of cannabis use on developing bodies. Some of Paton's work was criticized for inferring effects on humans from animal studies and for dosages being greater than those that would be found in cannabis smoking. But experimental pharmacology was largely focused on animal experiments, and Paton was a proponent of research on animals, highlighting their continued value to science throughout his career.[94]

Paton was troubled by the way in which pharmacological knowledge was utilized in the formation of policy. He was concerned by the inconsistency of the science–policy transfer: for example, the way in which knowledge could be applied to policy in respect to different drugs, such as in the case of cyclamates, DDT, and barbiturates. As he argued: 'One might venture a naive pharmacological comment on the odd fact that cyclamates are being banned never having done any damage to any human and only with difficulty to animals, while in millions of bathroom cupboards there lie ... lethal or near lethal doses of barbiturates.'[95] The inconsistent treatment of different licit and illicit drugs has remained controversial to this day.

Paton argued that for the formation of reputable policy there needed to be consistent criteria by which to assess substances – criteria that seemed to be non-existent. A few years later he reiterated the point that there seemed a split between the treatment of products developed through industrial processes – such as DDT and saccharin, which were coming under attack as dangerous products – and natural products like cannabis, which many argued was not dangerous.[96]

Paton also questioned where responsibility lay for all drugs, whether medical or recreational. Attitudes towards the mechanism of control of cannabis could swing between paternalism and permissiveness. For Paton, one way to avoid these extremes was to rely on accepted principles of public health and social legislation: for a drug to be made available it needed to meet criteria similar to those used for medicine or food additives, and its risks needed to be taken into account, as well as the number of consumers vulnerable to them.[97] Though Paton was not involved in some of the main expert committees of the ACMD in the 1970s, he tried to influence the public debate on cannabis and called for a precautionary approach to cannabis-related legislation. In 1978 he published an article on the impact of laboratory research on social policy. Drug policy, he argued, was made up of evidence and attitudes welded together. The article used cannabis as a case study and considered the interrelationship between science, medicine, and policy. He saw policy decisions around cannabis as critical because he believed that they had the potential to set a precedent for the treatment of other substances: 'It was with such a background that those interested in preventive medicine must consider the question of control of cannabis … One must ask whether a government would successfully control any chemical again, if it approved for general distribution a chemical substance known to be cumulative, found to be teratogenic in three species and possessing a wide variety of biochemical and cytotoxic actions.'[98] Unlike many proponents of decriminalization, Paton attempted to draw distinctions between cannabis and other substances such as tobacco and alcohol. He considered cannabis to be more dangerous than alcohol on the grounds that alcohol was ingested and was therefore not an irritant; additionally, it was usually ingested with food and was less cumulative. In contrast, he noted that cannabis was inhaled for its intoxicant effect, often diluted with tobacco, and it could result in non-obvious intoxication; it also had a serious toxicology dossier, with an unknown chronic dose level.[99] But it was difficult to apply consistent criteria when cannabis's role in the body remained unclear.

A key question in pharmacology is that of pharmacodynamics: the explanation of how a body interacts with a drug. Understanding the mechanism of action of drugs was important because it helped to explain the workings of the body, e.g. through the role of receptor systems. But in the 1970s the mechanism of action of cannabis was not yet understood. Paton had previously worked on the mode of action of anaesthetics, and he had argued that they were non-specific in action, making a detailed case for the properties of fat soluble (lipophilic) substances.[100] In seeking the mechanism of action of cannabis, Paton predicted that active principles such as THC, which were also fat soluble, had a resemblance to the anaesthetics. Pertwee in turn found that THC mimicked the anaesthetics, which seemed to support Paton's hypothesis. It was thought that this would account for some of cannabis's actions, such as hypotension, depression of cortical activity, and analgesia. This led Paton to consider that cannabis, like the anaesthetics, was also non-specific in action.

Paton's findings led Gill and another member of the team, D.K. Lawrence, to argue that there was no 'goodness of fit' for a specific cannabinoid receptor and that the mode of action was quite different.[101] This hypothesis moved research away from the idea of the specific action of cannabinoids and the idea that cannabis acted through receptors. Mechoulam later attributed this interpretation to an impure THC supply and commented on the impact of issues in the supply chain for cannabis research: 'A very prominent group in Oxford ... had done some work on cannabis, and ... thought that its activity was not specific ... It was based on some work with ... synthesized THC which was not very pure ... so Bill Paton thought maybe these compounds act non-specifically ... This was accepted ... It turned out there was a mistake in the chemistry ... The people who had synthesised it [had] ... not obtained very pure material ... that blocked investigation for almost twenty years.'[102] This avenue of research was not reopened until the late 1980s, when the hypothesis was disproved and a new understanding of cannabis's mode of action reopened the cannabis field, changing people's knowledge of how cannabis could act as a specific therapeutic.

PATON AND THE THERAPEUTIC USE OF CANNABIS

Paton's concerns over the potential harms of cannabis contributed to his disinclination to use it as a therapeutic: he argued in 1968 that he would 'defend the case that there is no valid therapeutic use for cannabis'.[103] He was sceptical about the anecdotal reports of cannabis's medical value. While both ancient and nineteenth-century uses of cannabis were often cited to support claims for therapeutic applications, Paton rationalized that, with so few drugs available, anything that offered hope was seized upon. Furthermore, cannabis as a therapeutic lacked clinical trial evidence, and for Paton this meant that cannabis had no contemporary proof of value.[104] But despite clinical trials being the route to drug testing and licensing, large-scale trials on cannabis would not take place for decades. Paton argued that there were more potent and more specific modern drugs to employ:

> Today it is proposed as an analgesic, antidepressant, hypnotic ... diuretic or antibiotic, for treating glaucoma ... psychiatric aid or treatment of withdrawal symptoms. For each of these uses there are more potent modern drugs. It is of greater significance that its modern rivals are also more specific ... Even though cannabis or THC has some particular action, its therapeutic use entails the production [of] tachycardia, conjunctivas, psychic changes ... or depression, euphoria ... Its fat solubility and pharmacokinetic properties too present difficulties for sustained use, although if its toxicity were acceptable, methods could be devised for dealing with these, as with other drugs.[105]

Paton viewed the apparent non-specificity of cannabis with its widespread effects as a problem and a limiting factor for any medical application. In later years, as will be discussed in the following chapters, this breadth of effects would be seen as advantageous.

The issue of medical cannabis became politicized by the mid-1970s. Potential medical use became caught up in campaigns for decriminalization. Lester Grinspoon, an American psychiatrist, became an early activist for medical cannabis and he wrote *Marihuana Reconsidered,* in which he illustrated anecdotal reports of cannabis's value as a medicine. In stark contrast to Paton he downplayed cannabis's dangers. Grinspoon had previously taken an anti-cannabis stance but, when his son, who suffered from cancer, found cannabis alleviated the symptoms of the chemotherapy, he became an advocate of legalization. This case and others like it raised the profile of cannabis for its therapeutic potential, highlighting the need for legal flexibility to cater for patients who had no other recourse. This triggered a response from anti-decriminalization scientists such as Gabriel Nahas, an anaesthetist pharmacologist at Columbia University in the United States. Paton and Nahas were united in their concern over the pressure for legalization. Nahas feared popular opinion was shifting against the precautionary principle: 'I am sure that it will take a good deal of time to dispel the widely spread new myth that marihuana is less toxic than alcohol or cigarettes.'[106] He stressed his fears: 'All these observations seem to have been performed a little too late in order to offset the momentum of the attractive but completely erroneous claims of Charles Kaplan and Grinspoon. I believe their claims correspond exactly to what many people want to hear today.'[107]

Paton agreed with the aim of Nahas's *Keep off the Grass,* and he contributed the book's foreword, in which he argued that 'the innocuousness of cannabis is being overstated and its dangers underestimated.'[108] Despite some differences of opinion, Paton was pleased to see this kind of work appear.[109] But the book did not sell well.[110] Popular texts on the anecdotal benefits of cannabis seemed to receive greater publicity and find a greater market. Indeed, problems with publishing cannabis texts dogged Paton.[111] Furthermore, Gill recalled that 'by the time we got to the middle of the 1970s ... there was no overwhelming case that could be made against cannabis on the grounds of toxicity. It was at that point that the subject lost momentum.'[112] Gill argued that Paton took an asymmetrical view of cannabis literature: 'He applied all his very considerable skills to a lot of what you might call the positive evidence (ie that it was not harmful) and was much more tolerant about the negative evidence.'

Paton and Nahas feared that the claims of therapeutic use would override research that suggested harmful effects in humans. Paton found cannabis useful for providing hints towards synthesizing related molecules because of its interesting structure but not as a medicine in its own right.[113] In his comments to a publisher on Mechoulam's idea for a new book on the therapeutic uses of cannabis in 1980, Paton argued that, in light of cannabis's somewhat scattergun impact on the body, it was useful only as a lead: 'There is ... a tendency ... to show that cannabis ... is therapeutically useful instead of ... trying to use the hints it provides to produce some really exceptional remedies by synthesizing related molecules. My own view is that the only therapeutic use of significance so far is as an anti-emetic in cancer therapy. Its effect in glaucoma and in bronchodilation and with cannabidiol in epilepsy ... aren't really useful as they stand ... The significance therefore I take to be potential rather than actual for the most part.'[114]

Paton did not completely condemn cannabis as a medicine, because he assumed it would be possible to deal with its cumulative problems if its toxicity was regarded as acceptable, as was the case with other medical drugs.[115] He wrote to Mechoulam about the link between therapeutic cannabis and politics: 'I was surprised that nabilone is being excluded from further trial ... I still think THC points to something interesting and exploitable but it's all bedeviled by politics and the pot lobby's desire for THC to be the winner.'[116] In 1983 he commented further on the dilemma: 'If your view is that it is harmless then the psychic effects and general somatic effect which would appear as side actions get discounted. If on the other hand its action and its cumulative potential have worried you in recreational use then they continued to do so in therapeutic use.'[117] For Paton there was a considerable gap between cannabis's potential therapeutic use and the advisability of using it as such.

CONCLUSION

At the time when cannabis research re-emerged, cannabis fell under the administration of both controlled drugs and the regulation of licit medicines. But when cannabis tincture was removed as a licit medicine in 1973, cannabis was left firmly in the arena of illicit drug regulation. While this move might have seemed to have ended cannabis's career as a medical substance, pressure to obtain a better understanding of cannabis as a controlled drug indirectly opened the door to remedicalization.

The isolation and synthesis of THC, the main psychoactive principle of cannabis, removed a hindrance that had stunted cannabis's use as a pharmaceutical product, and it permitted cannabis research to develop in a way that had not previously been possible. Interest originated from different scientific communities: sociologists and psychiatrists seeking to establish the epidemiology and the impact on mental and social health. Experimental pharmacologists like Paton investigated these compounds for physiological activity and demonstrated various effects of cannabis. Research was mainly animal-based laboratory work. It confirmed that THC was the main psychoactive constituent but that there were a number of other previously unknown active constituents. Other significant findings indicated that cannabis could interact with other drugs, had potential toxic effects, and could have cumulative effects because of its fat-solubility.

Research was hindered by supply issues in this period. Although problems were partially overcome, this drew attention to the difficulties encountered when there was limited industry involvement and no domestic supply. The quality of supply could be crucial in influencing research and the interpretation of research results, which in turn influenced developments within the field. The lack of an independent domestic supply and industrial involvement were issues that would have to be revisited in later decades.

Nonetheless, the background knowledge of cannabis that would allow therapeutic applications to develop in later decades was explored in this period. As Paton himself explained: 'There is a misunderstanding of the role of "basic" laboratory work. This may, if one is lucky, yield results with immediate application. But its real function is longer term, to provide the background knowledge and understanding and the rational framework in which opportunities for practical advance can be created and grasped.'[118]

By the mid-1970s many of the main chemistry and pharmacological questions had been answered. It was the interpretation of pharmacological findings in animals that was important, because it raised concerns over the possible effects in humans, and it appeared to give credence to earlier vague fears over the harms to individuals and to society, especially over mental health and the long-term effects for young users.

In this period science and policy became increasingly interlinked, and Paton articulated concerns to the scientific community, the public, and policymakers. The interpretation of results from laboratory work that used animals led Paton to campaign vigorously against the recreational use of cannabis. He emphasized the need to apply the precautionary principle in relation to cannabis, and he pressed for preventative approaches to cannabis by maintaining the status quo around existing legislation. However, he also raised the need for flexibility in the mechanism of drug control, to allow for changes in knowledge.

Through international science networks Paton was aware of research into therapeutic use, such as that by Mechoulam for glaucoma and epilepsy, and he did acknowledge that cannabis could be useful as a palliative in the treatment of cancer through chemotherapy. Overall, although Paton denied cannabis's usefulness as a medicine due to its potential long-term toxic effects and the possible resulting encouragement of recreational use, he did concede its potential usefulness as a lead.

Paton's laboratory research had put into place the building blocks that would allow research into cannabis's medical applications to progress. Paton, in a discussion of the importance of pharmacology, explained: 'Pharmacology studies the response of biological systems and their control by chemical substances with the special aim of improving therapeutics. Pharmacology underpins the pharmaceutical industry.'[119] With cannabis's basic pharmacology better understood, other pharmacologists began to write more positively about the drug, and, as is discussed in the next chapter, clinical pharmacologists, clinicians, and the pharmaceutical industry were now in a better position to begin to study cannabis's therapeutic applications.

Cannabis in the Clinic:
Clinical Pharmacology and
the Therapeutic Applications
of Cannabis, 1973–82

The interest of the medical profession is slowly reviving. It is not impossible that a limited but respectable niche will be established for it [cannabis] in therapeutics by the end of the century.[1]

While Paton wrote on the potential harms of cannabis, a change in attitudes towards cannabis among some pharmacologists became discernible. Clinical pharmacologists began to emphasize potential therapeutic applications and to question the interpretation of its harms. This chapter focuses on the role of clinical pharmacology through the work of J.D.P. Graham, and it traces the emergence of potential therapeutic applications of cannabis for glaucoma and epilepsy, its use as a pre-anaesthetic, and its use as an anti-nausea drug in cancer chemotherapy. I demonstrate how forces of necessity in the clinic led to some degree of acceptance of cannabis as a therapeutic. In particular, the application of cannabis as a palliative for the treatment of nausea caused by chemotherapy provided stimulus and legitimacy to the cannabis field.

But while previous cannabis therapeutics had focused on cannabis extracts in tincture form, the 1970s saw a very different focus on the form and the delivery system used to confer cannabis's therapeutic properties. After the removal of cannabis tincture's PLR in 1973, cannabis therapeutics focused on synthetic, single chemical entities, which attempted to improve on the active principle of cannabis in order to increase its efficacy and to reduce its psychoactive effect. A few small-scale clinical trials were carried out on versions of

THC, some of which made the leap through the regulatory processes in the United States and the United Kingdom. Within ten years of cannabis being removed as a medicine in the United Kingdom, the argument that cannabis had no medical value was being overturned, as emergent synthetic cannabis-based drugs were licensed for limited use in the United Kingdom and the United States. In contrast, investigations into smoked cannabis acted as a lightning rod for controversies over cannabis, herbal medicines, and smoking. Interest in cannabis's therapeutic potential had infiltrated policy discussions by the 1980s, with debates focusing on its benefits versus its harms.

Cannabis in the clinic posed serious problems for the drug scheduling systems. Over this period medical cannabis remained deeply interlinked with discussion around recreational use, but the need for new drugs in the clinic meant that cannabis as a medicine was forced into policy discussions. Despite advances in drug development, the newly introduced licit cannabis-based drugs were poorly tolerated by patients, and they were not widely marketed as a result of the stigma around cannabis and its placement within drug control systems. By the end of this period public health focus began to shift away from cannabis to other illicit drugs; with no development in the understanding of cannabis's mode of action, the field began to contract.

INTERNATIONAL RESEARCH AND THE THERAPEUTIC USE OF CANNABIS

While some experimental pharmacologists such as Paton concentrated on the harms of cannabis as demonstrated in animal studies, clinical pharmacologists started to investigate cannabis's potential in the clinic. Furthermore, with the chemistry of cannabis now better understood, both pharmaceutical firms and academic laboratories began projects on cannabis-based drugs.[2] Two areas opened up for cannabis therapeutics: one utilized the psychologic effects of cannabis, including its application as a sedative, analgesic, pre-anaesthetic, and anti-emetic; the other avoided the psychologic impacts and focused on cannabis as a bronchodilator, as an anticonvulsant, and also in intraocular pressure (IOP) reduction and tumour growth reduction.[3]

As is discussed in chapter 6, patient pressure in the United States encouraged research into cannabis for glaucoma.[4] Glaucoma is a condition of the eye in which the channels through which the fluid flows gradually become blocked and the IOP gradually builds, causing damage to the optic nerve and a gradual deterioration of vision. Standard treatments were limited. Emergent reports of cannabis's benefit for treating glaucoma were largely anecdotal, but some scientific research began. Hepler and Frank found that cannabis smoking reduced IOPs in normal subjects for four to five hours, and that there were no indications of serious side effects.[5] They concluded that cannabis might be more useful than conventional medication because it worked by a different mechanism. Hepler later found that when cannabis was smoked for months at a time by glaucoma patients, the effect on IOP stayed constant and there was no deterioration of vision.[6] Mechoulam was particularly keen to push work on the therapeutic applications of cannabis in glaucoma.[7] He had some success with local applications of THC on rabbits for glaucoma, and he wrote to Paton in 1976 about his research on cannabis and glaucoma as well as cannabis and epilepsy: 'We have gone ahead with the glaucoma thing but unfortunately although we have very good results in rabbits, we have no idea what relevance our work has for humans ... We are doing a double-blind clinical experiment with cannabidiol on epileptics with results so far much better than expected.'[8]

Yet it was difficult to transfer research into the clinical environment due to a dearth of toxicity trials on cannabis and THC. Mechoulam's project hit snags similar to those that had plagued Paton and the MRC in the early 1970s: it was unable to secure industry involvement due to the costs involved. Mechoulam complained to Paton: 'Industrial companies do not consider a new glaucoma drug worth the enormous expense of introducing it into the market so we are stuck!'[9] While researchers demonstrated some potential applications of cannabis and THC, only a few seemed worthy of research and development, especially for a 'controlled' substance. Paton, for one, was not convinced about the application of cannabis for glaucoma. He responded to Mechoulam that he found it had interesting cellular effects but that the interest was mainly focused on the impact on IOP and that people tended to miss the link with changes in blood pressure.[10] The National Eye Institute in the United States supported research studies from 1978 to 1984 in an effort to determine whether cannabis, or drugs derived from cannabis, might be effective as a treatment for glaucoma. The studies demonstrated that some derivatives of cannabis lowered IOP when they were administered but that there were also undesirable side effects, and that they did not compete favourably with other available drugs.[11] Research also emerged on cannabis as an analgesic, though reports were inconsistent, revealing a narrow window between beneficial and adverse effects.[12]

Rather it was as a drug in the management of cancer where cannabis's benefits were perceived to outweigh its harms and to justify involvement in cannabis-based drug development. It was this application that contributed most to cannabis's remedicalization during this period. The side effects of cancer chemotherapy presented a distressing problem, with new cytotoxic drugs such as paclitaxel (Taxol) causing nausea and vomiting, sometimes to the extent that the treatment was viewed as worse than the disease.[13] In some cases patients were forced to stop treatment. In the 1970s it was a relatively new but increasing problem. Available cancer chemotherapy palliatives were unsatisfactory. Phenothiazine was used but its benefits diminished with use and it had unwanted side effects. Other treatments, such as metoclopramide, were often ineffective. Since it was a clinically induced problem, and one that seriously limited the viability of chemotherapy as a tool, it was critical to find a solution.

Anecdotal observations of cancer patients in the United States had revealed that patients who used illicit herbal cannabis were less troubled by chemotherapy. Herbal cannabis, however, was in no way considered a suitable therapeutic, and chemists attempted to improve the efficiency of cannabis constituents by molecular manipulation, aiming to retain the activities of THC while removing the undesirable side effects. Mead has argued that attempts to divert patient pressure from herbal cannabis in the United States during the 1970s led to research funded by the National Cancer Institute, part of the NIH, on both smoked herbal cannabis and THC. Pre-clinical and clinical research was carried out into THC delivered in tablet form.[14] Sallan et al. have reported on trials with THC capsules given to twenty patients before and after chemotherapy, fourteen of whom found their nausea symptoms were alleviated.[15] Chang et al. have demonstrated that THC was superior to a placebo, and other experiments have shown that it was equivalent to, if not better than, other available treatments.[16] This is not to say that it was without side effects, some of which appeared worse than competitive drugs to clinicians, but patients seemed to prefer it. Six US states began trials that involved 748 patients who smoked cannabis and 345 patients who took THC capsules. These trials indicated that smoked herbal cannabis could alleviate symptoms of nausea and vomiting following cancer chemotherapy.[17] Legal restrictions made further research difficult, but popular pressure led twenty-one states to legislate to permit its use with cancer chemotherapy. Mechoulam, for one, was enthusiastic about this application and viewed it as a 'real blessing' for chemotherapy patients, pointing out that others found it to be the drug of choice.[18] These early experiments filtered through to British researchers.

CLINICAL PHARMACOLOGY: J.D.P. GRAHAM
AND THE THERAPEUTIC USE OF CANNABIS

One notable UK pharmacologist with an interest in the clinical applications of cannabis was Professor J.D.P. Graham. Graham had qualified in medicine and had developed an interest in the pharmacology of the autonomic nervous system during his time at the Nuffield Institute of Medical Research in Oxford. After war service he moved to Glasgow and later to Cardiff as a senior lecturer in pharmacology and a lecturer in toxicology, later becoming professor of pharmacology at the Welsh National School of Medicine in Cardiff. He wrote extensively on the pharmacology of therapeutics and on toxicology. He became secretary of the British Pharmacological Society in 1961 at a time when the society was expanding, and in his role there he sought deeper links with the pharmaceutical industry. A clinical section of the British Pharmacological Society was established in 1970 and the Society introduced a new specialist publication, the *British Journal of Clinical Pharmacology*, in 1974. This was important because the discipline of clinical pharmacology linked the laboratory and the clinic, and it assisted in the re-evaluation of cannabis as a therapeutic.

Throughout the 1970s and 1980s Graham published on pharmacology, as well as on the effects of cannabis on the respiratory and cardiovascular systems, and on its potential as a medicine in those fields.[19] He became an influential figure in both pharmacology and policy circles through his involvement in advisory committees. He became important to the process of remedicalization not only for his research but also for his advocacy of cannabis therapeutics within policy circles. One obituary in 1990 summarized his approach to life: 'Typically Scottish down-to-earth approach to everybody and everything but very much his own person, not intimidated nor daunted by obstacles or difficulties but clear and decisive in pursuing the path he saw to be right.'[20]

Graham's interest in the central nervous system led to work on narcotic analgesics, hallucinogens, and drug dependence. Early work had led to structural activity profiles of a-adrenoceptor blocking agents, antihistamines, and cannabinoids.[21] By the time he moved to Cardiff he had a particular interest in the effects of THC. Graham and his group worked by way of an MRC grant on the physiological effects of extracts of cannabis and THC, and they studied the cardiovascular and respiratory effects of cannabis.[22] Initial experiments by Graham focused on the cardiovascular effects of cannabis extracts and purified constituents of cannabis on laboratory animals, including cats and rats.[23] Experiments focused on tinctures of cannabis, produced by William Ransom & Sons, from which researchers extracted THC. Makor Chemicals also provided THC itself. Results appeared to demonstrate the ability of THC to reduce systematic blood pressure, pulse, and respiratory rate. Other constituents, including CBN and CBD, were found to have no effect on rats.

Graham went on to investigate the impact of cannabis on human subjects in the clinic. Respiratory diseases, including bronchial asthma, which had a rising fatality rate, were a growing problem. Early concepts of asthma as a psychosomatic disease had been overturned during the 1960s, and the condition became viewed as a disease with a physical component. Asthma was shown to have an inflammatory component, and the search thus began for drugs to treat the inflammation.

Pharmacology – and particularly autonomic pharmacology – had become a strong field in Britain, and it was important in the development of bronchodilators.[24] The medication isoprenaline had been used to treat asthma, but it had cardiac side effects, and the benefits were short-lived. Other treatments included barbiturates, but more effective, less harmful treatments were sought. The British medication salbutamol (Ventolin), an analogue of isoprenaline, was introduced in 1968.[25] Many of the effective therapies for asthma originally derived from natural substances, so it was not implausible to consider cannabis as a therapeutic.[26] Furthermore, unlike glaucoma, asthma had a high death rate, so there was pressure for the development of alternative treatments.

Research in the United States had shown that cannabis could cause an increase in the volume of the bronchial tubes. In the United Kingdom Davies and Weatherstone (from the Chest Disease Research Unit at Sully Hospital in the Vale of Glamorgan), Griffiths (from the Department of Psychological Medicine at the Welsh National School of Medicine, Cardiff), and Graham carried out small-scale, double-blind clinical trials on ten volunteer asthmatic in-patients, providing them with a placebo, THC, or salbutamol. The study revealed that THC and salbutamol significantly improved the patients' ventilatory function. The delivery method chosen for THC was via a metered dose by pressured aerosol, a new route of administration for THC. Nebulizers had been developed at the turn of the century using aqueous solutions, but they were superseded in the mid-1950s by the pressurized metered-dose inhaler.[27] By this method researchers found that THC was effective in an amount too small to alter mood or to be detectable by radioimmunoassay. In 1976, when they published the results of the study, they concluded that THC had potential as an adjuvant medicine for asthmatics.[28] Its novel mode of action meant that it had potential: 'The mode of action of THC differs from that of sympathomimetic drugs, and it, or a derivative, may make a suitable adjuvant in the treatment of selected asthmatics.'[29]

The bronchodilation effect of THC had gained international acceptance as a potential area for cannabis therapeutics by the mid-1970s. A 1977 United Nations Office on Drugs and Crime (UNODC) review written by Nahas, who was usually more noted for his opposition to cannabis, acknowledged research in this area and accepted that it provided a novel approach, though he concluded that there were problems with the method of delivery and potential side effects.[30] When Graham reviewed the work on the bronchodilator actions of cannabis for Mechoulam's book *Cannabinoids as Therapeutic Agents* in 1982, he was able to conclude that cannabinoids had a different effect from other bronchodilators.[31] He found that other constituents of cannabis had effects similar to THC, with few cardiovascular or psychological effects, though CBN and CBD were ineffective. In contrast, inhaled THC caused an increase in airway conductance, increasing the lungs' capacity to absorb oxygen.[32] Although this application for cannabis did not develop to the same extent as the application of cannabis for anti-nausea, the development of new delivery methods was important in the process of the remedicalization of cannabis. Developments in metered-dose, oral-mucosal sprays by the British pharmaceutical industry in later decades would prove important for the delivery of cannabis extracts.

Cannabis-derived anti-emetics were another aspect of Graham's work. Earlier reports of cannabis's psychic and somatic effects, combined with numerous anecdotal reports of the effect of smoked cannabis, meant that it was seen as having potential benefits for patients with incurable diseases, such as bronchogenic carcinoma, who were undergoing radiation therapy, which caused distressing side effects. Pilot single-blind clinical trials took place on patients who had inoperable bronchogenic carcinoma and who were suffering distress from radiation treatment. Two groups of six patients on a crossover pattern were investigated. Patients were administered oral THC or a placebo. Records of mood, sleep, pain, temperature, and cardiovascular parameters were kept. The study found that THC caused drowsiness, improved sleep, reduced pain, reduced elation and vigour, and increased fatigue and confusion. It also caused slight tachycardia and hypotension, as did the placebo.[33] Overall it was concluded that the aim to determine whether or not THC could be given readily and safely in a hospital setting and to establish an active but not toxic dose had been achieved, and it was found that 'the management of stressful patients was considered to have been improved by the drug'.[34] It was also seen as having wider implications for additional therapies: 'The state of passivity and relaxation shown in the above patients suggests that the anodyne (a medicine that relieves pain) may find a place in the management of patients undergoing psychologically disturbing therapy or investigation.'[35] With cannabis showing potential as an anti-emetic and being able to ameliorate distressing medical treatments, Graham went on to publicize the results of this research.

Graham was a good communicator and was keen to take the research on cannabis to a wider audience. His research in the 1970s led him to take a more positive and pragmatic approach to cannabis. Though he agreed with Paton that cannabis had toxic properties, he played down the dangers of toxicity and the drug's ability to cause dependence. He published two books on cannabis. *Cannabis and Health* was an edited collection published in 1976, for which Paton wrote the introduction. The book included a chapter titled 'If cannabis was a new drug' in which Graham compared cannabis with other available licit medicines. He argued that all medical drugs

had their individual problems and that cannabis was not unique in
that respect. He pointed out that other important plant-based medicines, such as aspirin and digitalis, would not have made it to trial
if they had been investigated in the 1970s.[36] In the text he drew attention to the revival of interest from the medical profession and
he foresaw a time when cannabis might operate as a niche drug. He
argued that approaches to drugs needed to be flexible in order to
take account of changing evidence. He pointed out the fact that it
was never wise to consider any drug to be permanently established
as a therapeutic, and he cited the experience of thalidomide and
also of rauwolfia, an evergreen tree from which an antihyperten-
sive drug is made. As a clinical pharmacologist he was keen for trials
to take place, arguing that scientific evidence was changeable, and
with that in mind he argued that sufficient research had been carried out to justify trials on cannabinoids: 'Insofar as the medical use
of cannabis is concerned a submission would be perfectly feasible in
so far as it applied to individual cannabinoid chemicals which can
be produced synthetically from precursors which do not involve cultivation of the plant, in a pure form to which quality control can be
applied ... Most of the work for THC has been completed ... There
is no reason now to deny a clinical trial certificate for a single chemical.'[37] Cannabis therapeutics, however, remained closely linked to
discussion of recreational use.

Arguments took place over the position of cannabis in society,
in particular its legal implications. Graham waded into this debate
when he wrote *Cannabis Now*, published in 1977. Graham took a
rather more relaxed view about occasional, moderate use of recreational cannabis. In his book, published for a non-specialist
audience, he reviewed the current state of knowledge about cannabis, the history of social responses to cannabis, and the debates
over its legal status. The book generally received favourable reviews.
Graham expounded his understanding of cannabis, arguing that it
did not cause physical dependence:[38] 'It is not a drug which causes
physical dependence and only rarely is it likely to cause a complete
desire for it, but one can readily become more than a little fond
of it.'[39] He accepted Paton's evidence that it could remain in the
body for some time, but he regarded its moderate recreational use
as less of a problem: 'Moderate smoking is not likely to damage
the brain or destroy the personality of the smoker but it would be
preferable to confine the habit to the weekends as cannabinoids

linger in the body.'[40] Graham deemed moderation, rather than prohibition and abstention, a more appropriate approach – a factor he
brought into policy discussions.

Berridge has described the two strands of public health that co-
existed in the 1970s and beyond: abstention was the line that Paton
took in relation to drug use; and risk reduction, which became
known as harm reduction and moderation of substance use, was the
approach favoured by Graham.[41] Intent on rehabilitating cannabis
as a therapeutic, Graham tried to draw the medical use of cannabis
away from the recreational debate. In his opinion, it was not cannabis per se that was dangerous, simply people's utilization of it. This
interpretation was similar in some ways to Paton's early query about
proposed drug control legislation: was it more feasible to control
the use or the administration of a drug rather than the drug itself?

Graham did not agree with the idea that the medical use of a
drug should be denied because it might drive recreational drug misuse, arguing that misuse of a drug was not a reason to withhold
trials: 'Highly accumulative drugs such as digitalis are used therapeutically, admittedly the need for this drug digitalis is urgent,
there are no alternatives ... It is by no means certain that THC will
not prove to be uniquely useful as it is distinctly unusual in its actions ... A trials certificate is not usually withheld from a new drug
of promise because there is potential for danger if people mishan-
dle the drug.'[42] Graham saw the potential benefits of the new drug
for mitigating diseases that lacked effective treatments as outweigh-
ing either the dangers of its side effects or its potential for misuse.
He posed the question of whether the scientific community was being ultra-cautious and, through fears of misuse, was failing to take
an opportunity to discover a potentially unique medicine that had
novel actions.

These views were important because Graham brought them into
the policy discussions of the 1970s and 1980s. These policy discussions are considered in detail in chapter 4, but it is important to
note that during this period governmental expert groups were set
up to advise on cannabis, and the divisions within the relevant scientific communities were played out within this policy framework.
These committees were significant for the process of remedicalization as they provided an early arena for discussion on the therapeutic
use of cannabis. They gave Graham a platform to influence the debate over policy. Graham became a member of the ACMD from its

inception in 1972 until he resigned in 1984. While Paton had been at pains to argue for the legal status quo, Graham had a different philosophical approach to the discussions surrounding the law, and he took a very different view of the implications of toxicity.[43] He was cautious in accepting the right of the government to impose legal restrictions on its citizens in that he felt that people should have more freedom to make up their own minds on such issues. Within the ACMD he downplayed the dangers of cannabis, brought therapeutics into the discussion, and pressed to make changes to the law.[44] His attitude led to heated discussions in the committee.[45]

As well as being influenced by the needs of his patients, his pragmatic approach and his desire for immediate action rather than retaining the status quo were other significant factors. His desire to get things done was reflected in his committee work on cannabis, in which he pressed members to be more proactive in making decisions based on available evidence rather than merely calling for more research and, as a consequence, delaying any decision-making.[46] Significantly, arguments by Graham and others facilitated initial attempts to draw the discussion of cannabis therapeutics away from concerns over the misuse of drugs. This move created an environment that was more receptive to the remedicalization of cannabis. Cannabis's therapeutic potential was an inconvenience to drug control policy, and it meant that in later decades attempts would be made to disassociate the two concepts and encouragement would be given to the development of licit CBMs.

Around this time mainstream medicine started to take more note of cannabis therapeutics. An editorial in *The Lancet* published in 1975 considered the therapeutic potential of cannabinoids, and Graham's work was referenced. Though the article indicated problems, and also doubts about some of the research, including the development of tolerance to THC, it raised the profile of cannabis as a legitimate therapeutic possibility. The pharmacological properties that were highlighted included sedative, analgesic, anticonvulsant, hypothermic, and hypotensive effects, as well as the stimulation of appetite, the lowering of intraocular tension, the relaxation of smooth muscles, and immunosuppressive actions. The article concluded: 'THC or more probably some derivative may well find a place as an adjuvant to isoprenaline, since the action on bronchial smooth muscle differs from that of isoprenaline, or as an anodyne in the management of terminal carcinoma.'[47]

The attitudes of some international organizations also showed signs of a shift. Both the UNODC and the NIDA, two agencies noted more for their hostility to cannabis, acknowledged cannabis therapeutics.[48] But throughout the 1970s medical use remained largely interlinked with concerns over recreational use, and this impeded remedicalization. A UNODC report from 1977 illustrated the fears: 'If marijuana products are proven to be useful therapeutic agents, their usefulness might well be attenuated if marijuana is widely used as a recreational drug.'[49] The report did, however, note that THC might be useful in the treatment of asthma and glaucoma and that CBD might be useful for epilepsy. NIDA was more positive: a report published in 1976 summarized contemporary research on cannabis and, in a section specifically concerning the therapeutic use of cannabis, indicated areas of potential interest and the fact that further study was worthwhile.[50] Possible applications that were noted in the NIDA report included cannabis for use in glaucoma and to aid bronchodilation. Particular benefits of cannabis therapeutics were described: the cannabinoid configuration, which provided a wide safety margin between effective and lethal doses; and, crucially, the mechanism of action, which appeared to differ from known mechanisms.[51] This different mechanism of action would become critical for the process of remedicalizing cannabis.

The concept of therapeutic cannabis was therefore back on the research agenda, but it took a breakthrough in laboratory research and in understanding the mechanism of action to reinvigorate the process of remedicalization. In the meantime, practical difficulties and controversies remained.

FORM AND DELIVERY: SMOKED HERBAL CANNABIS OR CANNABIS-BASED DERIVATIVES

Once the potential of cannabis as a medicine had been established, the question by the 1980s was what form the cannabis should be used in: would it be one single active principle, a synthesized version, or a herbal form; or was it only valuable as a lead for further investigations?

Paton's correspondence has revealed differences of approach between different researchers within the scientific community. Frances Ames, a South African neurologist and psychiatrist who researched cannabis using animals, found that baboons refused an extract of cannabis, forcing her to work with herbal cannabis, a concept which appealed to her.[52] Mechoulam experimented with both extracts and synthetic compounds. But on the whole there was more acceptance of cannabis derivatives than of herbal cannabis or of its extracts. Herbal smoked cannabis was rejected due to two concerns: its effect as an irritant and the properties of smoke.

Focus was shifted to specific cannabinoids and the ability of chemists to modify them. In the United States, NIDA suggested that active cannabinoids could be improved and that it should be possible to remove the psychoactive element and to provide a longer shelf life. The development of synthetic derivatives without the psychoactive element – and administering them through methods other than smoking – had the advantage of separating therapeutic cannabis from recreational cannabis. From NIDA's point of view there was no interest in moving cannabis or its derivatives through the drug control Schedules until they had passed through the regulatory processes of the US Food and Drug Administration (FDA).[53]

In the United Kingdom the reports of cannabis's, and THC's, anti-emetic properties stimulated a new avenue of clinical research; a handful of doctors applied for, and received, licences to investigate cannabis for this use in the early 1980s. On the whole, research focused mainly on the provision of cannabis in the form of oral THC. Clinical researchers included Professor J.S. Malpas from St Bartholomew's Hospital, Dr Speed and Dr Smith from the Royal Marsden Hospital, Dr J. Pritchard from Great Ormond Street Hospital, and Professor J.W. Thompson, a pharmacologist from Newcastle University, all of whom were licensed to administer oral THC.

Interest also arose in researching herbal cannabis. But it was far from straightforward to carry out such cannabis research, especially in a clinical environment. Clinical application was controversial, not only due to the continued linkage to recreational cannabis use but also for technical reasons: the trialling of herbal cannabis was contentious because the method of administration was via smoking. Cannabis smoke was considered to contain many carcinogenic substances similar to those in tobacco smoke, and there was increasing opposition to smoking. The BMA, for instance, would begin high-profile anti-smoking campaigns in 1984.

The experiments of Dr Michael Rose, a haematologist at St George's Hospital in Tooting and at St James' Hospital in Balham during the 1980s, illustrate some of the controversies of researching this form of cannabis in the clinic.[54] Rose was convinced that the investigation of cannabis derivatives and herbal cannabis was worthwhile. He applied for a licence to study oral trials of cannabis, but he later changed the application to include smoked cannabis. The discussion became political when Rose publicly complained that the legal situation constrained research, and he then placed public pressure on the Home Office to facilitate research. In an article in *The Lancet* in 1980 Rose argued that it was time to bring cannabis back into the clinic, especially in relation to cancer: 'There seems to be a population of cancer patients who may benefit from treatment with cannabis derivatives … This is a pressing and important area for research. Yet, currently the Home Secretary has issued only one or two licences for prescription of cannabis or its derivatives. I believe that failure to give cannabis to patients on cytotoxic therapy could be considered a matter of professional negligence.'[55]

For Rose, cannabis research was a question for the medical profession, not the legal profession. In his view, any problems related to the mode of administration, such as when cannabis was smoked, were technical rather than social issues. Rose complained bitterly about the effect of policy on research and medicine: 'What seems to be at issue is neither the therapeutic value nor the detrimental reputation of cannabis which have been disputed since 1839 … It is the state of public affairs which is awry.'[56] He was irritated by the actions of the Department of Health and Social Security (DHSS), arguing that it was the department's interpretation of the law rather than the law itself that was the cause of the problems. He claimed that although the law allowed for research, problems originated from the negative attitude of the DHSS towards cannabis: 'The law in the Misuse of Drugs Act 1971 makes provision for the clinical administration of cannabis … The Department of Health meanwhile without authority implicitly repudiates the public evidence of clinical potential supported no doubt by such ex cathedra sources as the British National Formulary … in which cannabis is dismissed as having no valid medical use.'[57]

According to the MDA, licences for research on cannabis had to be obtained from the Home Office. Rose's application to the Home Office was approved after the agreement of the DHSS. The DHSS agreed to permit the use of a room at St James' Hospital for the treatment to take place, and cannabis derived from the plant extract was obtained from the government chemist. But in practice it proved difficult to carry out the research. Licences took time to obtain and there remained the issue of cannabis supply. Rose became upset by what he perceived as hindrances to clinical research and, in particular, bureaucratic wrangling. After having battled through a complicated licensing system, he continued to criticize policy, and in 1981 he condemned the process in *The Lancet*: 'The licence was issued after almost six months of wrangling, pursued by florid attention in the press. Having issued the licence apparently under duress the Home Office disclaimed authority to provide the cannabis indicating officials at the Department of Health as a source of supply. They in turn put it blandly that ... release of cannabis for therapeutic purposes in the United Kingdom was more or less out of the question.' The DHSS responded that the question of therapeutic cannabis was under consideration and could not be answered in the interim. In the meantime, Rose's licence expired before he received any cannabis material.[58]

The issue of therapeutic cannabis in relation to such an emotive issue as the alleviation of chemotherapy side effects brought into question the precautionary principle. Rose questioned this approach in certain circumstances, arguing that the risk–benefit analysis was askew, at least in relation to cancer patients: 'Awaiting definitive conclusions, authorities behave with conviction that they are already available. Draconian regulation debars patients with intractable vomiting caused by chemotherapy from receiving cannabis as a potential source of relief. That seriously calls into question the claim that officialdom is acting with caution out of concern for the sick. These people are already bedevilled with problems: the calculation of risks and benefits must make allowance for their exceptional circumstances.'[59] Fears of cannabis toxicity and psychosis on which this precautionary principle was based were downplayed with some asperity by Rose: 'There is a disparity between the notable absence of danger associated with cannabis, and the behaviour of authority. The legions of insane, wrecked by their youthful ingestion of cannabis, are not exactly in evidence.'[60]

The exceptional circumstance generated by cancer chemotherapy drove a wedge into the precautionary principle and increased the pressure, particularly on the Home Office and the DHSS, to allow research. This put the DHSS in an awkward position. Even those individuals who had reservations or wished to take a more cautious approach towards cannabis considered that, in the light of constraints placed on cancer chemotherapy, the situation warranted further research. The debate continued in *The Lancet* when an editorial in 1981 observed the desperate need for new anti-emetics and acknowledged that, despite problems, cannabis-based drugs might have a role to play: 'An effective anti-emetic would revolutionize cancer chemotherapy ... There must be serious reservation about the use of a drug which produces alteration in mood and perception even if these applications are likely to be beneficial to some cancer patients ... Nevertheless, further studies on the anti-emetic properties of THC and related cannabis derivatives are desirable.'[61]

This editorial together with a clear need for additional medicines in the clinic sparked debate around the relative positions of potential medical drugs in the scheduling system. J.T. DuQuesne from the Psychopharmacology Research Committee in London questioned the positioning of cannabis with LSD and also the reasons for the discouragement of research. Writing in *The Lancet* in 1981 he acknowledged the need for research on cannabis: 'It is truly bizarre that cannabis is juxtaposed with lysergide (LSD) ... Whatever one's view of the possible adverse effect of cannabis, whether or not one believes, on the evidence, that it is habituating or holds other dangers, is it not absurd that Dr Rose and others are actively discouraged from undertaking serous clinical research, for example, such as may improve the quality of life for cancer sufferers?'[62]

These controversies were not unique to cannabis, however. Healy has shown how a number of drugs used in the field of psychiatry were feared because their social use was deemed to have political consequences. Controlled substances with therapeutic potential thus proved problematic. In the 1960s LSD also became increasingly prohibited and was in the same Schedule as cannabis in the United States.[63] Erika Dyck, for example, in her study on LSD and psychedelic psychiatry in the United States, has shown the complexities of dealing with a controlled substance that has therapeutic potential at a time of increasing alarm over drug abuse. In the case of cannabis, broader lay knowledge and the need for additional therapeutics called into question the existing policy on illicit drugs, in relation to both the inclusion and the position of drugs within the control system.

Public attacks on the system and reports appearing in *The Guardian* and *The Doctor* provoked concern within government departments, and pressure to defend government policy necessitated a note from the Chief Medical Officer to justify policy.[64] The note pointed out that cannabis was considered worthy of investigation and that four consultants in oncology held Home Office licences to evaluate the effects. It clarified the process whereby the Home Office referred to the DHSS for advice on the suitability of applicants to hold licences. Licences were granted by the Home Office on the recommendation of the DHSS, which established the doctors' credentials and the bona fide nature of their research. The Chief Medical Officer's response highlighted the problems of dealing with a drug that crossed the boundaries between a medical substance and a recreational one, and it also highlighted the likely cultural acceptance of cannabis in this instance. In relation to Dr Rose, the officials noted concerns over Rose but also the possibility of a public outcry if his licences were removed. They remarked: 'Officials do have some anxiety about Dr Rose and his activities but on balance it is felt that his present study is very limited and tightly controlled under Home Office regulations. There is a need to conduct studies of cannabis in patients with cancer and any move to revoke his Home Office licences would be counterproductive because of the inevitable emotive publicity this would generate. Dr Rose's activities will be closely monitored.'[65] *The Lancet* reported the position of the Minister of Health, Dr Gerard Vaughan, who had been forced to respond to Rose's complaints in September 1981: 'Dr Rose's original application to the HO was for oral trials but he later changed his research to include smoking cannabis ... The HO agreed to this but requested further information ... and evidence exists to indicate that smoking cannabis may be more carcinogenic than the smoking of tobacco ... The Department is not opposed to research into cannabis or its therapeutic potential but there are constraints under the law and a responsibility to avoid harmful side effects.'[66]

The method of administration was a key factor in the debate over the medical use of cannabis. It seemed that orally administered extracts of cannabis or synthetic THC in exceptional circumstances were acceptable, whereas smoked herbal cannabis was a step too far, especially in light of the anti-smoking campaigns prevalent at the time. Graham and Rose corresponded over the mode of administration of cannabis. Rose wondered if the aerosol method used in Graham's research with asthmatics would be transferable for anti-emetic purposes.[67] Developments in drug-delivery systems would indeed prove important for the process of remedicalization and were further developed in the 1990s.

The process of initiating trials was confusing for researchers such as Paton and Mechoulam. In 1981 Mechoulam wrote to Paton that he had several hundred grams of CBD but that he found it difficult to initiate trials for epilepsy, and he asked Paton if there were suitable groups in England that might be interested. Paton wrote to the Home Office, which forwarded the query to the DHSS.[68] The DHSS explained the system. There were two routes to research. The more usual system was for researchers to apply to the Home Office for a licence to possess and administer the drug. Such requests were then forwarded to the DHSS, who considered the suitability of the research worker and the project design before allowing licences to be issued by the Home Office. Alternatively, if the department wished to promote research in a particular field, suitable research workers would be informed and encouraged to submit protocols. But this route was for priority areas, and a demand for cannabis research had to come from the ACMD: 'Until the Minister has received recommendations of the Advisory Council regarding the priority of research into the therapeutic potential of cannabis the latter procedure could not be initiated.'[69] As is discussed in chapter 4, the ACMD did later give cautious consideration to the therapeutic benefits of cannabis, as growing acceptance of synthetic cannabis-based drugs offered greater legitimacy to the concept of cannabis as a medicine.

CANNABIS DERIVATIVES BECOME LICENSED MEDICINES

The urgent need to alleviate symptoms that were themselves being created by medical intervention meant that cannabis as a therapeutic was given a legitimate role. While researchers were able to carry out research on cannabinoids for various applications, bringing cannabinoids to patients on a large scale was another matter. Any CBM required a licence from the regulatory bodies, which were at that time the MCA in the United Kingdom and the FDA in the United States. Unlike the trials of cannabis for respiratory and cardiovascular problems that did not lead to a licensed medicine, the trials for the alleviation of symptoms caused by cancer chemotherapy led to licensing the production of cannabis-based drugs.

Synthetic THC presented the acceptable solution. A single chemical entity, orally administered version of THC was able to pass through regulatory systems in the United States and in the United

Kingdom. The pharmaceutical company Eli Lilly brought nabilone, an analogue of THC, to market, branded as Cesamet and targeted at cancer chemotherapy patients. As an analogue of THC it was hoped that nabilone would avoid the psychoactive properties of THC and the associated concerns over misuse.

The role of the pharmaceutical industry in bringing nabilone to market is detailed further in chapter 5, but the drug was licensed in 1982 for prescription-only, hospital-only use against nausea arising from chemotherapy in the United Kingdom, where patients were unresponsive to other treatment, and it was licensed in the United States by the FDA in 1985. It initially appeared to offer an acceptable way forward. Leslie Iverson, a pharmacologist with an interest in policy, later explained that clinical trials opened the door to two new drugs: 'The result of properly controlled clinical trials in the 1970s and 1980s indicated that the two cannabinoid drugs, dronabinol and nabilone, appeared to offer a potential important advance over the relative ineffective anti-sickness medicine available in the 1980s.'[70] A decade after the removal of all CBMs, cannabis derivatives based on THC, the active psychoactive principle of cannabis, were back in the medicine cabinet.

However, these new medical drugs quickly ran into a set of problems. Nabilone was not widely marketed and it was withdrawn in the United States in 1989, though it remained available in the United Kingdom and Canada. Dronabinol (Marinol), which was synthetic THC, was given approval by the FDA for the treatment of nausea in cancer chemotherapy in 1985. Marinol was never marketed in the United Kingdom. These derivatives had significant problems. The psychoactive effects, which could not be totally avoided, remained of concern to doctors and patients, and this constrained their application. Both derivatives proved unpopular with patients for several reasons, including the 'high' produced as a side effect and the time lag between administration and effect. In addition, use of the derivatives was heavily restricted due to fears over the potential diversion to recreational use. More effective, non-cannabis-based competitor drugs quickly emerged – ones that were soluble in water and were therefore usable as an intravenous (IV) injection at the time of therapy: a preferable administration method for patients with nausea. Furthermore, with no progress on the mode of action of cannabis, no one really understood how THC-based drugs worked. However, despite their problems and limited uptake, the arrival of

these synthetic cannabinoids in the clinic was critical for the process of remedicalization. It marked the reintroduction of licensed
CBMs and provided cannabis research with a degree of legitimacy,
which encouraged further investigation of cannabis from a therapeutic viewpoint rather than a continued focus on its deleterious
effects. It also left open the potential for research into herbal cannabis in later decades.

LOSS OF INTEREST IN THE CANNABIS FIELD

The sudden surge of interest in the pharmacology of cannabis that
had developed from the 1960s proved short-lived, and by the late
1970s and for most of the 1980s the field ceased to develop. Pertwee
described meetings of the British Pharmacological Society in which
cannabis was essentially ignored, with cannabis posters being rele-
gated to the sidelines and cannabis talks pushed to the last session
of the last day. He commented later: 'No one was interested. "Why
work on cannabis?" was a constant question. It got a bit depress-
ing.'[71] One problem was the absence of dedicated cannabis research
societies and the infrequent nature of relevant symposia, which
failed to motivate the discipline. Pertwee recalled: 'In the 1970s and
1980s there weren't any cannabis societies and there'd be the occasional symposia, but many of those were organised in a way that you
always had the same speakers. It was all very constrained … It wasn't
very encouraging for the development of the field.'[72] This was because work had become descriptive, centred on the chemistry and
the pharmacology, but without any advance in understanding the
mode of action there was little opportunity to carry out exciting new
research. Pertwee described the situation: 'We had run out of things
to do. Very descriptive, just describing the pharmacology. There was
no handle on the mode of action … All pharma was thinking about
cannabis and then abandoning it.'[73]

Understanding the mode of action was crucial for allowing cannabis research to proceed meaningfully. A report by NIDA in 1977
indicated the potential importance of discovering cannabis's mode
of action for research and medicine: 'In addition to the possibility
that therapeutic benefits may one day accrue another reason for
studying the potential medicinal value of the cannabinoids is the
possibility that their mechanism of action may be different from
the currently available medicaments. In this case the elucidation of

these mechanisms would be even more significant than the mere discovery of another therapeutic agent.'[74] In 1978 the MRC's Addiction Review Group concluded that: 'In view of the adequate amount of work on the pharmacology of addictive drugs there was no need to specifically encourage more in the future.'[75] Without a breakthrough in the mode of action, the cannabis field began to contract, as many researchers and funders switched to other areas of interest.

The cannabis threat was being superseded by other concerns, including 'hard' drugs such as cocaine and heroin and new public health fears over the emerging disease AIDS. Also, interest shifted away from drugs such as cannabis towards a greater focus on licit drugs, including alcohol and tobacco. By the 1980s comments in the House of Commons highlighted the economic and social costs of alcohol and tobacco as opposed to those from illegal drugs.[76] Pertwee recalled the shift and the impact of changing incentives for researchers: 'People were running out of things to do and the thing was winding down, people were leaving the field ... going into amphetamines, or dependence, or ecstasy ... other drugs of dependence. They couldn't get funding basically, on cannabinoids.'[77] Paton's analysis when he acted as a referee to Mechoulam's book *Cannabinoids as Therapeutic Agents* summed up the altered environment: 'One should resist the book being too long. I might add that I think there would be a reasonable but not enormous sale. I think the cannabis field is getting less fashionable.'[78] Thus, although the medical cannabis field had taken large steps forward, it had hit another substantial barrier.

Some individual researchers including Mechoulam and Pertwee maintained their own enduring interest in cannabis despite the general trend. This continued interest proved important for later developments in the cannabis arena. Pertwee later described his reasons to remain in a diminished field: 'I stuck with it and decided to develop this assay. I just felt it useful to have. Very lucky for me that the receptor was discovered and I could be in at an early stage.'[79]

Pertwee had moved from Oxford to Aberdeen to establish another research 'cell' in 1974.[80] For his research he drew on work in the opioid field. Hans Kosterlitz and his team, who were based in Aberdeen, became famous for their discovery of opioid receptors in the brain and the endogenous morphine-like substances that they termed enkephalins.[81] This discovery explained why opiates

worked. The discovery of the opioid receptor proved important for
the concept of addiction to borderline substances such as tobacco.
This research eventually provided the rationale for understanding how the brain deals with pain and enabled the production of
new analgesics.

The research techniques used by Kosterlitz were important for
cannabis research. Kosterlitz worked on opium using mouse vas
deferens.[82] Pertwee's experiments examined whether this process
could be applied as a bioassay in the cannabis field, and his research
later proved fortuitous as it turned out to be a sensitive assay for the
cannabis agonists that were developed later in the 1990s. As with the
discovery of opioid receptors, a breakthrough in cannabis's mode
of action and the discovery of cannabinoid receptors in the late
1980s would reawaken the cannabis field and open up new avenues
for cannabis research, as well as leading to new understandings of
how the human body functioned.

CONCLUSION

Within a decade of banning cannabis tincture, cannabis-based
drugs were back in the clinic. Research by clinical pharmacologists
had initiated more positive approaches to cannabis with discussion
of its potential therapeutic benefits. Numerous potential applications for cannabis as a medicine were investigated, but it was its uses
as a bronchodilator, as an anti-emetic (especially in the management of cancer), and for glaucoma that became the most widely
accepted avenues.

Focus was given not to 'whole cannabis' but to synthetic, single
chemical entities derived from cannabis, such as THC. These synthetic cannabis-based products reopened the therapeutic arena, as
they appeared to offer a way to improve the efficacy of cannabis
and at the same time reduce undesirable side effects. The search
for solutions to new clinical problems related to cancer chemotherapy saw the move from anecdotal to evidence-based medicine, with
the provision of larger-scale clinical trials. Some clinicians such as
Dr Rose pressed for the investigation of herbal cannabis, but the use
of smoked cannabis as the delivery method meant that the use of
herbal cannabis was interlaced with controversy.

Clinical pharmacologists like Graham expounded the potential
benefits and played down the dangers of cannabis use, bringing this

viewpoint to both policymakers and the public. Even researchers with a more cautious approach such as Paton and Nahas recognized the potential therapeutic avenues. As discussed in the next chapter, expert groups in the United Kingdom began to take note of the importance of this developing area, and it began to influence discussion around cannabis policy more generally. But the perceived interaction between medical and recreational use remained a major stumbling block to medical applications.

While sustained interest in cannabis therapeutics would not re-emerge until the late 1990s, the period between the mid-1970s and the late 1980s reawakened the concept of cannabis as a medicine and began to overturn the WHO's 1951 pronouncement that cannabis had no medicinal value. Importantly, while cannabis remained firmly routed in illicit drug regulation, cannabis derivatives through the involvement of the pharmaceutical industry re-entered the licit medical drug arena through the licensing of two cannabis-based drugs in the 1980s. As Paton had predicted, cannabis acted as a lead to other drugs and not as a drug in its own right. These, as pharmaceutically produced substances, entered drug control regulations and were still tightly controlled and rarely used. This left the door open to further CBM, and in particular to the investigation of herbal cannabis.

But just as knowledge of cannabis's medical properties was burgeoning, interest in cannabis from governments and funding bodies declined. It would take a breakthrough in the understanding of cannabis's mode of action in the 1990s, and subsequent sustained pharmaceutical industry involvement, to revitalize the cannabis field, leading to the next steps in the process of remedicalization and establishing CBMPs in the clinic. But for now, new knowledge in the clinic and the science–policy transfer of this work by clinical pharmacologists such as Graham helped create a policy atmosphere that was more favourable towards the concept of CBM.

Evidence-Based Policy?
The Development of Expert
Committees, 1972–82

During the time when research into cannabis and its therapeutic applications was emerging, moves to make policy more evidence-based were underway. This chapter traces the remedicalization of cannabis within the context of the development of expert advice. Historical research has shown that 'the idea of rationality, that there could be a rational relationship between research and policy, was high on the agenda' by the 1970s.[1] Berridge has demonstrated how this trend had an impact on dealing with both licit and illicit drugs, and has also shown where policy was in flux. She has revealed how this shift in government advisory mechanisms opened doors between government and professional bodies, allowing for interactions between specialists and policymakers. Evidence-based policy became the goal, emerging through a mechanism of expert committees that formalized informal networks of advice.

In the drugs field, previous ad hoc committees were reconstituted as the statutory ACMD in 1972 with the aim of providing advice to government on drugs of misuse. This mechanism of an institutionalized statutory expert committee became an important forum for policy discussion on cannabis. Around the time the ACMD sub-committees on cannabis were created, cannabis, which had previously come under the jurisdiction of both illicit drugs and licit medicines, lost its PLR and became solely aligned with drugs of misuse. However, as research re-emerged on cannabis's therapeutic use, the implications of the research were drawn into the discussions on drug control policy, and the expert committees became an early arena for discussing the therapeutic use of cannabis prior to the therapeutic-use-specific discussions and public reports of the 1990s.

Three significant deliberations are considered in this chapter. The first of these is the ACMD's Working Group on Cannabis (WGC), 1972–76, which discussed research gaps and legal issues and also produced two interim reports. It witnessed animated discussion between committee members over the relative harms of cannabis, and it contained the occasional reference to research on therapeutic cannabis.

The second committee to be studied is the reconvened ACMD's WGC, 1977–79, which focused on the impact of potential amendments to the MDA through proposed amendments to the Criminal Law Bill. The committee's discussions led to a decision to recommend the downgrading of cannabis from class B to class C. The decision was the outcome of heated and divisive debates over the position of cannabis in the control system and the relative dangers of cannabis.

The final committee that the chapter considers is the ACMD's Expert Group on the Effects of Cannabis (EGEC), 1980–82. This group had a new membership and was less acrimonious. It featured more prominent discussion of cannabis therapeutics, influenced in part by clinical trials of cannabis for the treatment of the side effects of cancer chemotherapy. When the EGEC released its report in 1982, it, too, recommended the downgrading of cannabis and the encouragement of research into cannabis as a medicine.[3]

This chapter considers how these expert groups were established, the influence of their membership, and the impact of therapeutic cannabis. It also tracks the evolving discussion over therapeutic cannabis within the broader drug policy debate.

THE ADVISORY COUNCIL ON THE MISUSE OF DRUGS AND THE WORKING GROUP ON CANNABIS, 1972–76

Historical and social science studies from the broader literature provide methods of looking at the role of expert advice that can be applied to the cannabis field. The term expert advice covers a variety of structures, as Barker and Peters have described, ranging from institutional civil servants and advisory committees to more informal information networks and contacts.[2] In the UK context, MacLeod has shown how the role of the professional and the expert developed in the mid-Victorian period,[3] while Hamlin has described how disputes flared between these experts.[4]

Expert advice evolved into a more formalized setting in the twentieth century, and Berridge, in her analysis of smoking policy in Britain, has discussed the development of advisory bodies or expert committees.[5] She placed deliberations over smoking in the context of developing relationships between experts and the state, along with the growing demand for the 'rational expertise-based model' within government, especially within the context of health policy and developments in the NHS. As Berridge has shown, the model of channelling scientific advice into policy was utilized in the illicit drugs field, and the formula was developed in detail during the 1970s with the formation of the ACMD.[6]

As will be discussed, it was during the 1960s that some of the initial expert committees were established in the illicit drugs field, on an ad hoc basis, and the 1970s saw the formation of statutory committees, which became deeply concerned with the cannabis question. The formal structure of an expert committee may be seen as one of the better ways of achieving evidence-based policy. For instance, Bulmer has shown how it provides a method of neutralizing a subject by taking it out of the political arena.[7] This is especially important with a highly divisive issue such as cannabis use. How far a committee can be successful in this is open to question. Cannabis never really escaped its politics.

During the 1950s and the 1960s, expert committees were established in the illicit drugs field on an ad hoc basis. This included the 1965 ACDD and its significant Sub-committee on Hallucinogens chaired by Baroness Wootton, a leading British sociologist and criminologist. This committee delved into the pharmacological, clinical, pathological, social, and legal aspects of these drugs and produced the Wootton Report in 1968, primarily focusing on cannabis. It raised issues that recurred in future debates, such as the relative harms of cannabis compared with other drugs, both licit and illicit, and it pressed for flexibility in the drug control system and questioned policies such as the police powers of stop and search.

Following the 1971 UN Convention on Psychotropic Substances, UK policy led to the MDA in 1971, which addressed the need for an ongoing specialist advisory body. The ACDD was reconfigured as a statutory body and renamed the ACMD. Its remit was to keep under review drugs that were being misused, or were likely to be misused, and to advise on measures that would prevent misuse or to deal with associated social problems. It returned to a number of questions raised by the Wootton Report.

Membership of the committee was by Home Office appointment. Ministers were obliged to consult the ACMD before laying Orders before Parliament or before making regulations under the MDA, though they did not have to act on its advice. This necessitated a working relationship between experts and government, but from its inception, the relationship was uneasy.

Cannabis was initially a major feature of the ACMD's work, and this proved to have consequences for remedicalization, since it would open the door to cannabis research. The WGC sub-group was created in 1972 to advise the Council. It met for the first time in December 1972, and between 1973 and 1976 it produced two interim reports. The WGC was established to consider facts relevant to the use of cannabis and other psychedelic drugs not normally in therapeutic use, and to examine the need for further research.[8] It was not tasked with reporting to ministers at this point but was set to provide the ACMD with a better understanding of cannabis in the context of growing international and domestic campaigns for a relaxation of controls on the drug. Cannabis's position in class B of the 1971 MDA had proved controversial and there were calls for decriminalization, either by changing the position of cannabis in the classes or by reducing associated penalties. Control measures that had emerged, such as stop and search, were particularly inflammatory and became a key area of debate for the WGC. But the evidence on which to formulate advice was limited, and in discussing control policy the issue of cannabis therapeutics arose.

The different professional backgrounds of the members meant that behind the WGC's reports lay mixed messages and different approaches to both the scientific evidence on cannabis and what to do with such evidence. The membership included Bob Searchfield, a social worker and director of the Standing Conference on Drug Abuse (later DrugScope); Griffith Edwards, director of the Addiction Research Unit at the Institute of Psychiatry; and J.D.P. Graham, a clinical pharmacologist who had worked on cannabis and who had sat on Wootton's Sub-committee on Hallucinogens. The WGC was chaired by J.C. Bloomfield, a pharmacist. Strong personalities emerged. Graham, influenced by his research, took a more benign view of cannabis and pushed its therapeutic aspects. He was keen to make recommendations for action. One obituary described his forthright personality: 'Jimmy was an energetic and forceful character. Always eager to get things done now ... He was frank and forthright, blunt even. And would become impatient and even on occasion impetuous when ... events were unnecessarily hindered by bureaucracy or more cautious individuals.'[9] Edwards later described Graham's approach as 'asymmetry personified – he believed that cannabis should be legalized'.[10] In contrast, Edwards was against liberalization, and he highlighted the potential harms of cannabis, preferring to maintain the legal status quo. These two figures symbolized the ongoing conflicts of the committee.

At its first meeting the group decided to consider the current literature on cannabis, cannabis's use within the United Kingdom, and the form of the debate on cannabis. Edwards attempted to introduce a framework by which cannabis could be assessed, and this informed many of the discussions. His 1973 paper to the committee, entitled 'Cannabis and the criteria for legalization of a currently prohibited recreational drug', identified criteria to be employed when deciding whether any drug should be legalized and then applied them to cannabis.[11] This placed discussion of cannabis within the context of not only the rise of regulatory frameworks controlling drugs but also increased control of food additives and a heightened awareness of previously underrated dangers of already accepted substances.[12] Within this context Edwards argued that the legalization of cannabis could not be justified. Instead, the question hinged on how cannabis could be prohibited without bringing the law into disrepute – a major problem with an illicit but borderline or peculiar substance, one whose position between being licit or illicit is negotiable, or one that can cross the line from being a widely consumed substance to a dangerous drug.[13] Attitudes varied. Searchfield was concerned with the social effects of penalties.[14] Edwards, although he recognized potential injustices, was more concerned with the long-term public health threat, which in his view necessitated a coercive legal framework.

The indeterminate nature of cannabis was reflected in the discourse of the working group. Though cannabis was classified as a drug of misuse, research both in the United Kingdom and abroad had begun to raise the question of whether cannabis should be viewed once again as a therapeutic drug, and the work of the broader scientific community entered into discussions. Graham brought various areas of research to the attention of members, including his own work on the physiological effects of cannabis extracts and THC, pharmacological work on cannabis and the immune response by W.D.M. Paton, and studies that had found cannabis to be an antipyretic (i.e. a drug that prevented or reduced fever).[15] While therapeutic cannabis had become more acceptable, its advisability was disputed because of perceived risks. Edwards took note of the therapeutic research in his 1973 paper, but he questioned where the balance between benefits and risks lay.[16]

The form in which cannabis might be utilized was an important issue. Splitting cannabis into its constituent parts was one method of moving remedicalization forward. Dr D.A. Cahal from the DHSS drew attention to the lack of standardization of herbal cannabis, but he argued that THC should be approached as would any new drug, and that if indications of therapeutic qualities existed then clinical trials should be carried out to test efficacy and safety.[17]

The WGC produced its first interim report in 1973, demonstrating the level of uncertainty around cannabis, the inability of the WGC (and therefore the ACMD) to provide expert advice, and thus the urgent need for further research.[18] Indeed, uncertainty has been crucial to the story of the remedicalization process. One important theme that emerges from the wider literature is the role of uncertainty in the decision-making and policymaking process.

Jasanoff, for example, in looking at the role of expert committees in the United States in relation to carcinogens in the 1970s and 1980s, has shown their growing importance to policymakers, and she has illustrated how the technocratic model is by no means value-free.[19] Her work considers what lies behind the construction of 'evidence' or expert advice, as well as the balancing acts between the costs and benefits of regulation: the 'trade-off between risks to health/environment and the economic/social costs of regulating'.[20] Jasanoff has demonstrated how scientific uncertainty could be used to influence policy.[21] This is particularly interesting in the case of cannabis, where uncertainty over its medical benefits and potential hazards were utilized by those on both sides of the debate.

Hilgartner, in a review of expert advice in relation to diet and cancer, has demonstrated how uncertainty could be invoked to justify action or inaction.[22] Hilgartner has also raised another issue: the role of private versus public discussions. Hilgartner likened the work of expert advice to the world of the theatre, with the performance (or report or publication) on view at the front of the stage, while backstage the actors (or in this case the experts) could discuss and rehearse their 'performance' in a private, enclosed space. Leaks blurring the division between this public and private space were viewed by Hilgartner as a breakdown in stage management. This approach is pertinent to the case of cannabis, where uncertainty, conflict, and leaks played key roles in the expert discussions of the 1970s.

Florin, in a review of the relationship between science and policy in terms of coronary heart disease prevention, aimed to assess the extent to which policy on health promotion in general practice was based on evidence.[23] She indicated that high levels of scientific uncertainty led to different interpretations of the evidence by those from different backgrounds. Overall, the wider literature has raised relevant questions for a study of cannabis: did uncertainty over cannabis's effects also have an impact within the framework of expert committees, and what impact did it have on advice and its uptake?

The WGC's interim report was approved by the ACMD and submitted to ministers, but calls for further research on cannabis created concerns within the ACMD and policy circles that the report, if made public, would boost calls for legalization.[24] These discussions were intended to be kept out of the public domain, an approach that was not unusual in the 1970s. Edwards and the chair were content to leave the report in the private arena, while Searchfield, who tended to be in favour of legalization, was keen to make the report public. Graham saw no problem with publication but did not make an issue of the point. The fear that the public might misunderstand the advice has been an often-repeated explanation of why the government has rejected expert advice on cannabis since the 1970s. Concern over social factors and wider debates over cannabis were certainly embedded in the members' discussions. Aspects of cannabis research were especially contentious, particularly experiments with smoked cannabis, because of the link to recreational use and the conflict with anti-smoking campaigns.[25]

In the end the report was not published. Nevertheless, the need for a clearer scientific base stimulated remedicalization because it opened the door to research. Arrangements were made for a further research sub-committee of the Interdepartmental Co-coordinating Committee on the Misuse of Drugs, which had been established to facilitate the work of the ACMD, to study the recommendations, and to take steps to effect them through the appropriate research council or by direct application to the Home Office or the DHSS.

Cannabis remained the focus of the second WGC report. Topics of discussion included how to obtain data on cannabis users, the police's stop and search powers,[26] and the effect of control measures.[27] Therapeutic use entered discussion to a greater degree, and the balance in the risk–benefit analysis began to shift. Graham argued that the drug's potential as a medicine outweighed any risks. A paper he presented to the WGC in 1975 highlighted cannabis's potential as a sedative, an analgesic, an appetite stimulant, an immunosuppressive, and a method of reducing IOP. Citing his own work at the Welsh National School of Medicine in Cardiff, he drew attention to the possible uses of cannabis for both asthma and cancer patients.[28] How cannabis should be utilized remained uncertain: Graham appeared to favour derivatives over herbal cannabis.

The main focus of the WGC was on control measures, however. The apparent failure of the criminal justice system brought drug policy into question, and the concept of decriminalization was gaining ground. The harms of cannabis had taken on a new meaning – they referred not to the pharmacological impact but rather to the social impact of controls. The WGC queried the aim of drug policy: was eradication still a possibility, or was the emphasis moving to discouraging new users and influencing the prevalence of use?[29] Division within the group intensified. Edwards expressed his general satisfaction with current laws. Searchfield reiterated his concern over the policy of fines and drew attention to the fact that the concept of decriminalization was finding support despite the prohibitive moves of international agencies.[30] There was no unanimity, and while the second interim report of 1975 recommended that there be no changes to the law in the light of uncertainty over the long-term clinical and social effects, it was accompanied by a minority report by Searchfield that favoured liberalization.[31]

The report was endorsed only in the expectation that the working group would reconvene within twelve months to continue its work and to yield more productive results.[32] The issue of penalties was referred to other discussions on the penal system in connection with a study of maximum sentences. The report was submitted to ministers but it was not published. The Home Office remained wary of reopening public debate and of risking the report becoming incorporated into calls for legalization.[33]

The report was not allowed to fade away quietly, however. Leaks had plagued the discussions, and private, closed discussions had found their way into the public domain. The debate over a loophole in the law relating to cannabis leaves and the stark divisions within the WGC were leaked to *The Guardian* and the *New Scientist,* as well as to Release, a voluntary drug organization set up to advise drug users about the law.[34] There were fears within the government and the ACMD that Release planned to publish an article and to quote from the report.[35]

The issue of leaks featured prominently in discussions during 1976. Searchfield, whose private correspondence was deemed responsible for the leaks, argued in favour of publication on the grounds that 'interest reflects the public interest and suggests that it was better to seek publication from the outset in order to deflect criticism'. Graham perceived that public interest in cannabis had diminished and that there was therefore reduced political sensitivity. For Graham this made it the appropriate time to discuss the issue, though in his opinion publication was only worthwhile if the working group drew conclusions. Others, like Philip Myers, Chief Constable of the North Wales Constabulary, were afraid of reigniting the controversy. D. Turner, a civil servant from the Home Office, focused on the role of an expert group being to advise, not to court public opinion. Edwards was against publication generally.[36] Concerns were raised not merely over the leaks themselves, but over the fact that they were targeted at Release, an organization associated with legalization. G.I. de Deney of the Home Office drugs branch linked the leaks to Searchfield: 'Release is an organization which does a lot of good work. But it argues for legalization ... Alarming the second interim report should have found its way to this organization ... Suspicion must, I'm afraid, attach fairly strongly to Mr Searchfield.'[37] The ACMD remained against publication, citing the fact that the report was an interim report, not a final one, and that the cost of publication was an issue, especially in the light of the report's limited conclusions.[38]

In sum, between 1972 and 1976 expert discussion began as an exercise in information gathering. Discussions revealed the paucity of the knowledge base on which to ground policy and added pressure for research. Although reference was made to therapeutic cannabis, the main impact was to encourage cannabis research, which would later indirectly lead to therapeutic applications. While government was looking for expert advice, existing evidence remained debatable, and as such it became an issue of interpretation leading to division among members. With no clear conclusions, further research and maintenance of the legal status quo was recommended, and the report was never published.

THE WORKING GROUP ON CANNABIS, 1977-79

The WGC did not reconvene again until 1977, when it was asked to advise ministers on potential changes to the 1971 MDA through amendments to a criminal law bill. The amendments, if adopted, would remove from the MDA the power of the courts to impose custodial sentences on summary conviction for unlawful possession of cannabis.[39] The ACMD advised a delay pending its re-evaluation of the general principles that governed the control of drugs and the application of those principles to various offences around controlled drugs.[40] The issue was the position of cannabis in either class B or class C of Schedule II of the 1971 MDA, as opposed to the issue of legalization.

Three ACMD sub-committees were asked to consider the question. The Technical Working Group chaired by Graham considered scheduling in relation to the pharmacological properties of cannabis and harm when misused. Another working group considered legal and administrative matters, and the WGC, chaired by Bloomfield, considered the question of scheduling more broadly. In 1979 the ACMD, on the advice of its working groups, published its decision that cannabis and cannabis resin should be downgraded from class B to class C and from Schedule I of the regulations to Schedule II.

This recommendation to ministers by the ACMD was not based on unequivocal advice from its working groups. A report by the ACMD in the 1980s summarized the conflicts around the need to act in the face of uncertainty: 'Some members' appraisal of all the available scientific evidence so far leads them to conclude that some alleviation of the penalties for unlawful possession could be contemplated ... Others having regard to ... inconclusive scientific investigation are not satisfied that enough is known to make recommendations which would widely be regarded as implying that the risks of using cannabis and cannabis resin are less serious than was believed.'[41] Scientific uncertainty meant that the evidence was open to interpretation and that policy imperatives differed for each member.

Divisions were most clearly demonstrated in the WGC's 1977 discussions in relation to the different stances taken by Edwards and Graham over the harms of cannabis use and the resultant policy. Graham, in his paper on the long-term effects of cannabis on health, questioned the validity of the data on harms,[42] and as chair of the technical sub-committee he called for the transfer of cannabis derivatives to less restrictive Schedules.[43] Doubts about the harms of cannabis use brought the criminal justice system into question. On these grounds the WGC recommended downgrading.[44] However, this initial decision to downgrade was quickly challenged because Edwards, who had been absent at the critical meeting, disagreed with both the interpretation of the evidence on harms of cannabis use and what that meant for policy. In correspondence with the chair, he explained: 'I would not myself have felt able to support those recommendations and was rather surprised to hear that the recommendations seem to have been made in the light of an impression that there is no evidence that cannabis can damage health … My own belief [is] that the scientific evidence which has been accumulating over the last few years goes rather in the direction of suggesting that cannabis may well be a much more dangerous substance than … had previously been supposed.'[45]

In Edwards's view the uncertainty over harms necessitated the retention of the precautionary principle and justified the maintenance of the legal status quo. At the following meeting, he argued that the committee's decision should be based not 'on proving harm, but the possibility of harm'.[46] Bloomfield, swayed by Edwards's argument, now argued that the law protected first offenders from imprisonment and there was therefore no reason to change the penalties. In addition, he feared that problems might arise from public misunderstandings if there were changes to policy.[47] The resultant split in the committee proved difficult to resolve.

In a statement that illustrated how different professional standpoints can influence expert committees, Edwards argued that Graham's approach to the problem differed from his own because Graham came from a pharmacological background whereas his own approach was epidemiological. Furthermore, in his opinion it was a question not only of evidence and its interpretation but also of the role of the committee, the legal system, and the government. Graham commented: 'It was merely a question of attitudes. If one was paternalistic, which he was not, then one felt justified in stopping people harming themselves.'[48]

The practicalities of downgrading cannabis further highlighted this conflict in approach. Edwards was concerned that cutting penalties for possession but not for supply was illogical. Additionally, he believed that the law had a part to play in educating people to realize that the use of all chemicals carried risks and that it would therefore be best to leave the law as it stood. Graham countered that this was not the role of the criminal justice system.[49]

In the end, cannabis was split into its constituent parts. The sub-committees concluded that THC was a dangerous substance and there were no recommendations to remove this from class A. This was not the case with herbal cannabis, as evidence of harm remained inconclusive.[50] The final report stated that a deterrent was still needed but that cannabis should be transferred from class B to class C and that the penalty of imprisonment on summary conviction for unlawful possession of all drugs in class C should no longer be available.[51]

But what would the government make of the expert advice? The ACMD's advice was rejected by Merlyn Rees, the Home Secretary. Dr D.J. Hardwick from the Ministry of Health wrote to members of the ACMD justifying this, not on scientific grounds, but on the need to retain the deterrent effect.[52] The report generated a degree of public interest and the Legalise Cannabis Campaign (LCC) quickly published 'Trash Rehashed', which criticized the ACMD for not going far enough.[53] It also raised the issue of access to cannabis for medical purposes on prescription.

In summary, between 1977 and 1979 a change was discernible. Though discussion of cannabis became increasingly acrimonious, in general the dangers of cannabis were played down, and the ACMD recommended downgrading cannabis from class B to class C. While the recommendations were ultimately rejected by the government, cannabis harms were called into question and the WGC adopted a more relaxed attitude to cannabis.

THE EXPERT GROUP ON THE EFFECTS OF CANNABIS, 1980–82

The EGEC was established in 1980 when the ACMD wanted to consider the scientific basis for the control of cannabis under the 1971 MDA.[54] This time the expert group was chaired by Graham. He continued to bring the issue of therapeutic cannabis into a more prominent position in discussions. The group included many of the previous committees' members, including Bloomfield and Edwards. Other members included Professor W. Cranston from St Thomas' Hospital; Dr B. Hunt from the DHSS; Dr G.P. McNicol, principal and vice-chancellor of the University of Aberdeen; Mr D. Turner, from St Bartholomew's Hospital; Dr B. Saunders and Dr D.J. Harvey from the department of pharmacology at the University of Oxford; and, at the request of Edwards, Sir W.D.M. Paton, who had worked for many years on cannabis.[55]

For the first time the issue of the medical use of cannabis was specifically raised in the remit of this expert group: 'If the appropriate bodies decided that cannabis had value as a therapeutic agent it would be possible to amend the regulation to authorize doctors to use cannabis.'[56] The use of cannabis for the alleviation of symptoms caused by the chemotherapeutic treatment of cancer had forced the issue. This movement of cannabis into the clinical environment caused concern as it blurred the boundary between an illicit drug and a licit one. It was viewed as risky to prohibit access to cannabis in such circumstances as it was assumed that there was sympathy in the wider community. Therefore, the ACMD set up this expert sub-committee in April 1980 to evaluate the therapeutic use of cannabis.[57]

The wider environment around medical cannabis was shifting. By the 1980s the WHO was retreating from its stance that cannabis medicine was obsolete and moving towards a cautious acceptance of cannabis's medical utility.[58] In the United Kingdom, while the earlier advisory committees had discussed the relative benefits or harms of therapeutic aspects of cannabis, by the 1980s the focus shifted to the technical issues surrounding such research. Even at the DHSS there was interest, and Hunt presented on the therapeutic use of cannabis to the expert group. He highlighted the many avenues that had been investigated and reiterated that the most promising application was as an anti-emetic for patients undergoing cancer chemotherapy.[59] The debate had moved on from one focused on the advisability of CBM to one focused on safety and efficacy: 'The efficacy of cannabis as an anti-emetic was undeniable, but it could be questioned whether its efficacy outweighed [its] toxicity.'[60] However, the dangers were not considered to be great enough to discourage research, even on additional applications such as epilepsy, asthma, and glaucoma.[61]

The final report of the EGEC was significant for the remedicalization of cannabis. Firstly, the report placed the burden of proof on proving the harmful effects of cannabis, which it argued had not been fully demonstrated: 'There is insufficient evidence to reach any intestable conclusions on the effect of cannabis on the human body, it affirmed that research undertaken so far failed to demonstrate positive and significant harmful effects on man solely due to the use of cannabis, and that areas where evidence suggested deleterious effects needed further research.'[62]

Secondly, the issue of therapeutics had become important enough to warrant specific discussion and recommendations. Importantly, the report acknowledged that scientific study had endorsed anecdotal reports of cannabis's medical applications, and it indicated a need for further research: 'Its use as an anti-emetic in cancer chemotherapy appears to be most promising and other possible therapeutic uses are in relation to glaucoma, epilepsy, and muscle spasticity, but much more research is required before its use in any of these areas can be accepted as a standard method of treatment.'[63]

These conclusions provided some legitimacy for therapeutic cannabis, and the report considered how potential CBMs could be made available. The regulations allowed for amendments to the MDA of 1971, and it was possible that cannabis could be shifted from Schedule I to Schedule II of the MDA regulations, which would permit research and medical uses.

In relation to cannabis control, the expert group recommended the downgrading of cannabis from class B to class C and reiterated that the penalty of imprisonment on summary conviction for unlawful possession of cannabis should be removed. Again, its advice was rejected by government, not on the evidence but on the message it gave.[64] Fear remained over potential 'misunderstanding', and a draft press release deleted the following sentence: 'Much of the research has failed to demonstrate the positive and significant harmful effects in man attributed solely to the use of cannabis.' It did, however, refer to the evidence suggesting that the therapeutic use of cannabis 'may after further research prove beneficial'.[65]

In 1982 a meeting on the therapeutic use of cannabis was arranged to clarify where, within the DHSS, responsibility for policy on therapeutic cannabis should lie. Dr Wrighton from the MRC argued that, if the use of more powerful cytotoxic drugs continued to increase, cannabis would become more interesting to UK researchers. The law was not seen as a deterrent to research; rather it was the cost and the supply of THC, which no UK firm was prepared to synthesize, that were the problem. Furthermore, a product licence for manufacture had to be obtained but could not be granted prior to the Committee on the Safety of Medicines being satisfied with safety. This meant that clinical research had to be repeated in the United Kingdom before CBMs could be made available. To facilitate this, it was agreed that attempts should be made to encourage researchers to apply to the MRC with protocols that provided the costs of THC. A policy split between medical use and misuse was encouraged within the DHSS.[66] But by this time the focus on cannabis in research and policy circles was shifting away to other drugs of misuse.

In summary, the 1980–82 period saw less heated discussion and less focus on cannabis harms. Specific discussion on therapeutic use emerged, and research into therapeutic applications, rather than research into cannabis generally, was encouraged. With cannabis derivatives entering the clinic, therapeutic cannabis was accepted as a potential reality, and discussion focused less on the wisdom of using it as a medicine and more on the cost and practicality of doing so. The public health needs of cannabis as a therapeutic had become more influential in driving discussion. Recommendations to downgrade cannabis were again rejected, but penalties were, in effect, reduced.

CONCLUSION

Expert advice and science–policy transfer proved critical in the remedicalization of cannabis. Early on, the discourse took place in the closed expert committees of the ACMD. The transfer of science to policy was enabled by the developing mechanism of expert advice via expert committees and the desire to place policy on a strong evidence base, especially in the illicit drugs field. Cannabis's borderline position and widespread use within the community necessitated significant discussion.

The drugs problem had been framed under the criminal justice system but, as the limitations of this were revealed and as other pressures mounted, both from the focus on civil liberty and from the practicalities of implementing a penal approach, new approaches were sought. As cannabis functioned as a medical product in self-help circles and as a potential medicine in the laboratory and the clinic, policy was becoming out of step with scientific developments and the issue of therapeutic cannabis was increasingly drawn into policy discussion, providing a route for science–policy transfer.

However, the science on which to base advice and policy was by no means clear. Cannabis extracts like THC had only just been discovered, the mode of action remained unknown, and the nature of evidence over relative harms and therapeutic use shifted over this period. The reports and archival material of these early committees highlight these issues of uncertainty and the changing nature of evidence. Uncertainty, not only over knowledge of cannabis's uses but also over what to do with the 'evidence', allowed for subjective decision-making within the WGC and allowed the government to decide whether to take or ignore its advice.

With uncertainty being a critical factor in discussions, it allowed the discourse to be influenced by key individuals from different scientific disciplines. Graham, a clinical pharmacologist, was able to question the evidence on harms, and in light of his own research he pushed the potential benefits for patients, while Edwards, a psychiatrist, was much more concerned with possible harms and any long-term threat to society. Not only was their scientific analysis of the evidence different, but also they brought different social values to the problem, e.g. on the function of the law.

As Jasanoff has shown, the 'evidence' of expert committees can be socially constructed and is not value-free.[67] Due to the discussions being on a politically sensitive issue, external pressures, such as the media and the decriminalization-of-recreational-use debate, compounded these conflicts. Creating a rational relationship between science and policy and focusing purely on the evidence proved difficult in practice. The committees were certainly well aware of the potential impact of their advice, as highlighted by the issue of leaks, which were both feared and utilized as a mechanism to open up debate. Controversies over the remit, membership, operation, and transparency of the ACMD would flare again in the early 2000s.

Although the advice in relation to the classification of cannabis was rejected by government, the process of science–policy transfer and the professionalization of expert advice created a slightly more flexible and relaxed attitude towards cannabis within the policy network. The highlighting of uncertainty around cannabis and the need for more research on which to base policy opened the door to further cannabis research. Uncertainty did not disappear, but it was this combination of more relaxed attitudes towards cannabis, research incentives, and the developing need to draw medical uses away from discussion of drug control that enabled remedicalization to develop.

In this period the issue of therapeutic cannabis was not yet disassociated from discussion of recreational use and control measures, as it would become in the 1990s to a degree. When by the end of the 1980s a breakthrough in the mode of understanding of cannabis emerged, cannabis as a medicine would become treated as a topic in its own right, and it would provide the justification to split cannabis as a medicine from discussion over the control of recreational cannabis use. Practical hindrances to cannabis research would be considered by the specific, independent, public therapeutic committees that emerged in the 1990s, which paved the way for clinical trials and UK pharmaceutical involvement in medical cannabis. This provision of pharmaceutical-grade medicinal cannabis would go some way towards causing the split between recreational and medical cannabis that was deemed necessary by policymakers.

4

Industrializing Cannabis:
The Pharmaceutical Industry
and the Remedicalization
of Cannabis, 1973–2001

The pharmaceutical industry has been crucial in the process of the remedicalization of cannabis, and this chapter charts the gradually increasing interest from industry after the loss of cannabis tincture in 1973. This chapter overlaps slightly in time with other chapters but it provides an in-depth analysis of the role of the pharmaceutical industry in the process of remedicalization. It begins by describing the problems caused by a lack of industry interest pre-1973. In contrast, it then considers the importance of temporary industry involvement in the 1970s and the 1980s, which provided two boosts to remedicalization. Firstly, there was the development of compounds that never reached patients but were useful for scientific research; and secondly, there was the production of synthetic cannabinoids that entered the clinic and became licit, if unpopular, medicines.

From the 1990s, major scientific breakthroughs opened two new avenues of research and re-stimulated industry interest. One avenue was the investigation of drugs that could activate the newly discovered ECRS – drugs that were not based on cannabis itself – and the other was the investigation of extracts of cannabis. Nineteen ninety-seven marked the dawn of a new era when GW Pharmaceuticals, a small UK biotechnology company established solely to investigate herbal cannabis, began the cultivation of standardized cannabis plants to produce CBMEs that would be delivered via a new drug-delivery system. This chapter places the remedicalization of cannabis in these contexts: developments in the pharmaceutical industry and the rise of biotechnology; the interrelations between academic science and industry; the rise of phytomedicine; and the major scientific discovery of cannabis's mode of action via the ECRS.

CANNABIS IN THE LABORATORY:
THE PHARMACEUTICAL INDUSTRY
AND CANNABIS PRIOR TO 1980

In the twentieth century the history of therapeutics was inseparable from the rise of the pharmaceutical industry. Historical and sociological research provides frameworks for investigating the role played by the pharmaceutical industry. Histories of pharmacy and the pharmaceutical industry divide the industry's development into several stages: kitchen physic or home remedies; the rise of commercial remedies (often mixtures of secret ingredients); the development of pathology and microbiology; the growth of multinational pharmaceutical companies, acquisitions and mergers, and the elimination of small-scale industry; and the emergence of small biotechnology companies.[1]

These different stages of the pharmaceutical industry have been reflected in the process of the remedicalization of cannabis. In the initial development of the pharmaceutical industry, historians have cited the importance of a greater understanding of vegetable and mineral substances that were used as medicines.[2] The isolation of an active principle was essential. Major discoveries included the isolation of morphine from opium, aspirin from willow bark, and later quinine from cinchona. In the late nineteenth and early twentieth centuries, when these discoveries were being made, cannabis was more of a commercial remedy than a pharmaceutical-grade medicine. As discussed in chapter 2, its active principle was not discovered until 1964, and it was first synthesized in 1965. Cannabis missed the 'cascade of medicine' that took place during the 'therapeutic revolution' of the 1940s to 1960s, which led to the expansion of the pharmaceutical industry worldwide.[3] In the United Kingdom, the development of the NHS and its mass market for medicines stimulated a flurry of new drugs, such as cortisone, beta blockers, and the contraceptive pill. Aside from its technical problems, cannabis remained unattractive to the pharmaceutical industry as a result of its increasingly prohibitive legal status.

This dearth of interest from a flourishing pharmaceutical industry had wider implications for the understanding of cannabis: it caused problems for academic research. Authors who have written about the pharmaceutical industry and pharmacy have highlighted the importance of accessing research material and how it can shape social and cognitive developments. One of the major issues for research into cannabis pharmacology was the lack of a ready supply of the active principle, THC.[4] Industry was not interested in producing THC or developing CBMs. Mechoulam later explained how the legal status of cannabis deterred companies: 'Many of the major pharmaceutical companies ... had small groups working on cannabis. But as soon as it went up ... the bureaucratic ladder ... all ... decided not to go with cannabis because of the bad publicity. They were afraid of it.'[5]

Fleeting pharmaceutical-industry interest proved important. Reacting to reports in the 1970s that cannabis and THC suppressed pain in experimental models, an international pharmaceutical company, Pfizer, developed a synthetic cannabinoid compound called levonantradol, an analogue of THC, as a potential analgesic, as well as the related compound CP-55,940. These compounds proved more water soluble than THC and were therefore more useful for research purposes. Pfizer carried out pilot clinical trials with levonantradol in suppressing post-operative pain and in preventing the nausea and vomiting associated with cancer chemotherapy. However, unable to separate the beneficial clinical effects from the intoxicant effects, Pfizer had abandoned the project by 1980.[6]

Throughout most of the 1960s and 1970s industry interest remained focused on alternative directions or showed only fleeting attention. The pharmaceutical industry itself was facing increasing restraints on its operations and was undergoing a slowdown in development. Slinn has explained the impact on the production of new drugs: 'When that took place not only was the therapeutic revolution over, but increasing regulation to ensure product safety ... was making the time between the discovery of a new compound and its launch ... much lengthier, eating into patent life. The R&D process ... was ... becoming much more expensive.'[7]

However, while these compounds were abandoned by Pfizer as medical products, they later provided a useful tool for academic cannabis research.

CANNABIS IN THE CLINIC: THE DEVELOPMENT OF
SYNTHETIC CANNABIS-BASED MEDICINES, 1982–87

The 1980s heralded a major new development in the process of the remedicalization of cannabis. Pharmaceutical-industry involvement in the United States built on the 1970s research into cannabis-based drugs, and two cannabis-based drugs made it out of the laboratory, through medicine licensing systems, and into the clinic. The main interest from the pharmaceutical industry's perspective was to find compounds that had the benefits of cannabis but without the psychoactive element. Companies hoped that such products could circumvent the restrictive legislation around cannabis.

Eli Lilly and Company had prepared cannabis preparations with standardized tincture of cannabis indica in the early 1890s and went on to develop nabilone, a synthetic cannabinoid and an analogue of THC, in the 1980s. While nabilone was not a naturally occurring cannabinoid, it was pharmacologically very similar to phyto-THC. It was branded as Cesamet for prescription to cancer patients.[8] With no other effective treatments for nausea caused by chemotherapy, nabilone was approved in 1982 for hospital-only prescription for 'nausea and vomiting caused by cytotoxic chemotherapy unresponsive to conventional anti-emetics' in the United Kingdom, where it was not a controlled drug.[9] Cesamet capsules for the treatment of nausea and vomiting associated with chemotherapy were licensed by the FDA in 1985.[10]

Another cannabis-based drug was dronabinol, an isomer of THC. Unimed, a newly established subsidiary of the Belgium-based Solvay Pharmaceuticals, bought it from the National Cancer Institute, part of the NIH, in order to bring the drug to market.[11] Dronabinol, marketed as Marinol, received approval from the FDA for the treatment of nausea in cancer chemotherapy in 1985. By 1987 it was distributed by Roxane Laboratories, an independent subsidiary of the German corporation Boehringer Ingelheim; and later, in 1992, its approval was extended in the United States to cover appetite loss related to AIDS. Dronabinol (Marinol) was never licensed in the United Kingdom, though it could be prescribed as an unlicensed drug on a named-patient basis. These were the first cannabis-based drugs introduced to market since the removal of cannabis tincture.

These licit medical drugs faced two problems. Firstly, they proved unpopular with patients; and secondly, medical derivatives of cannabis posed problems for the drug control agencies, as they re-introduced a dual role for cannabis. In discussing the development of the 1971 Convention on Psychotropic Substances, McAllister has demonstrated that the pharmaceutical industry argued for a cost–benefit analysis of psychotropic substances, claiming that under medical supervision the benefits of psychotropic substances out-weighed their risks and that they therefore warranted less stringent control measures.[12]

These arguments did not seem to work for pharmaceutically produced derivatives of cannabis. The US Drug Enforcement Ad-ministration concluded that nabilone was too closely related to cannabis and gave it a Schedule II classification under the US Con-trolled Substances Act, signifying that the agency considered it a dangerous drug despite having some medical usefulness. With can-nabis as the lead compound, nabilone was not far enough removed from its source. This classification placed rigorous restrictions on the use of the drug.[13] Eli Lilly, upset by the strict classification, lost interest and never marketed it, although researchers in the United Kingdom did use nabilone for clinical research.[14] It was also expen-sive, and Eli Lilly discontinued it in 1989.[15]

In 1971 the UN Convention on Psychotropic drugs placed dron-abinol in Schedule I, and this placement proved problematic for its widespread use as a medicine product in the form of Marinol. In 1987 the US government requested that the UN transfer dronabinol to Schedule II of the 1971 Convention, and it also asked the WHO to consider the matter. The WHO, recognizing some therapeutic ben-efit in certain instances but also the close relationship to the plant, rated the abuse potential as 'high' but argued that dronabinol should be downgraded to Schedule II: 'The abuse liability of dron-abinol is high and its therapeutic usefulness [is] moderate to high ... Although few public health and social problems are currently associated with the therapeutic use of dronabinol, this substance is the active principle of cannabis and is capable of producing the same effects as the plant material.'[16] The decision was not unani-mous: two members of the WHO committee disagreed, fearing that downgrading dronabinol would send out the wrong message and would promote the abuse of cannabis and its extracts. While the medical agencies were demonstrating a shift in attitude and were looking at cannabis medicines more favourably, drug control agen-cies were not. The UN Commission on Narcotic Drugs concurred

with the minority view when it chose not to endorse the recommendation of the WHO committee, arguing that cannabis's benefits did
not outweigh its potential for abuse.

There was a dwindling number of new drugs in the pipeline in the
1970s and 1980s. There were several reasons for this. Drug discovery
had come to be based on an understanding of the underlying mechanism of disease: a process that took much longer than the accidental
discoveries of the past.[17] The spiralling cost of healthcare, an ageing
population, and the rise of chronic diseases encouraged governments
to demand lower prices for pharmaceuticals, which contributed to
the restructuring of the pharmaceutical industry in the 1980s.[18] Cannabis research declined as researchers who had been involved in the
1960s shifted their research interests to emerging drugs such as amphetamines and cocaine, and funding for cannabinoids dried up.[19] In
such an environment CBM might have remained dormant but for major discoveries that revitalized the whole field.

UNDERSTANDING CANNABIS'S MODE
OF ACTION AND THE ROLE OF THE
PHARMACEUTICAL INDUSTRY, 1988–97

After receptors were discovered … cannabis became respectable … Lots
of drug companies still worried about drugs that activate receptors so they
looked at blocking them … for example for blocking appetite … There
was lots of money to be made out of that.[20]

In the mid-1980s researchers questioned the lack of stereospecific-
ity of cannabinoids and began to hunt for specific receptors for the
psychoactive cannabinoids in the brain. By the late 1980s interdisciplinary international research between medicinal chemists and
pharmacologists working on cannabis yielded results that led to a
breakthrough in the understanding of the mechanism of action of
cannabis, thereby clarifying the way in which cannabinoids worked
on the human body. This research reopened the issue of cannabinoid receptors and led to the discovery of what is now known as
the endogenous cannabinoid receptor system (ECRS).[21] The interdisciplinary approach was vital. Steve Hill, a professor of molecular
pharmacology at Nottingham University, highlighted the importance of the interdisciplinary approach to pharmacology and the
discovery of drugs: 'The power of collaboration between chemistry

and pharmacology is immense and the success of this alliance has underpinned astonishing successes in the development of powerful therapeutic drugs.'[22] This interdisciplinary approach was particularly important in the process of the remedicalization of cannabis.

Pertwee has expressed the importance of developments in pharmacology, which provided an improved understanding of the mode of action of cannabis, e.g. signalling by G-protein-coupled receptors.[23] Chemical signalling is the primary means to control biological functions, and the role of the receptor is to recognize these chemical signals. Receptors are important in medicine; they are described as lying at the heart of pharmacology.[24] Targeting receptors had become a focus for modern drug technology, and research demonstrating that cannabis acted on receptors therefore proved pivotal to cannabis's remedicalization.

Developments within the pharmaceutical industry provided the tools that ensured that research on cannabis receptors could take place. This was a classic example of how industry could influence academic research.[25] The cannabinoid compounds abandoned by Pfizer were given a new lease of life in academic circles: they proved to be a better tool than THC for researchers. Pertwee later described the importance of the compounds: 'It was those compounds that led to the discovery of the receptor. THC although it does bind to the receptor is so fat soluble, it's very difficult to show that it binds. Can't actually use it as a probe.'[26]

By radiolabelling the Pfizer compound to act as a tracer, it was possible to detect the recognition sites of receptors.[27] It became almost certain that cannabinoids were specific in action and that they acted on a G-protein-coupled receptor, overturning Paton's original hypothesis that cannabis did not act on receptors. Dr Allyn Howlett, a pharmacologist at Saint Louis University School of Medicine, who had done post-doctoral research at the University of Virginia involving the characterization of the first G protein, along with Bill Devane, a graduate student at St Louis, published conclusive evidence in 1988 that cannabinoid receptors existed in the brain.[28] The cloning of the CB_1 receptor in the 1990s confirmed Howlett's discovery.[29] Developments in cloning thus confirmed evidence of a cannabis receptor. Pertwee described the interrelations between cloning and pharmacology: 'It was lucky the field was developing in parallel with these important advances … Cloning was really in … so once it was cloned that was it, the receptor must exist.'[30]

Receptor cloning became a major preoccupation of molecular pharmacologists and by 2000 pharmacology had entered a new era.[31] The distribution of CB_1 receptors, found predominantly on central and peripheral nerve terminals, accounted for characteristics described earlier by pharmacologists, as well as benefits described by patients in the 1970s and 1980s. A periphery receptor, CB_2, was a further receptor that was unexpectedly located by the US pharmaceutical firm Sterling Winthrop in the United Kingdom in 1993, when it was searching for an anti-inflammatory drug.[32] This discovery of a receptor outside the brain was important because it opened up the possibility of achieving a cannabis-like effect without the problems of cannabis, just as the pharmaceutical industry had tried to do with drugs like nabilone.[33]

These discoveries led to the next crucial questions. What was the role of this receptor system? Did the human body produce cannabinoid receptor agonists, chemicals that bind to the receptor, or did only the plant compounds affect the receptor?[34] Mechoulam's group provided the next piece of the jigsaw. Mechoulam theorized that there must be a chemical that originated in the body (endogenous) and he sought to identify it. He later commented: 'We assumed that these receptors are not found in our body because there is a plant out there but the brain forms some kind of compound that will activate these receptors when needed. So we started looking for these endogenous compounds.'[35]

This was a complex process involving international and interdisciplinary cooperation, technological advances, and serendipity. Devane moved to Israel to take up a post-doctoral position with Mechoulam, and there he searched for the assumed endogenous cannabinoid. Along with a Czech researcher, Luis Hanus, Devane synthesized a new radioactive probe, which the pair used to help identify the substance. They extracted a promising candidate from a pig brain. Once they had material that seemed pure, they utilized the advanced techniques of nuclear magnetic resonance spectroscopy to establish the final structure of an endogenous cannabinoid, later termed anandamide. Recent technological advances had made these discoveries possible, as Mechoulam later elaborated: 'When we isolated anandamide ... we had essentially nothing, we barely saw the material we isolated but the machines were happy with it ... [This] couldn't have been done twenty years earlier.'[36]

Technological developments in the field made it possible to work with much smaller amounts of material and to considerably speed up research. Rang, in a history of receptors, has explained the importance of such technological developments: 'It took a full year to make the binding measurements, carry out the necessary controls and estimate the binding parameters – a task now routinely performed by a technician in less than a day.'[37]

It was necessary to establish whether this potential substance could activate the CB_1 receptor, but Mechoulam's group lacked sufficient material to carry out the tests. Others within the cannabis network provided the solution. Pertwee's decision to stay in the cannabis field and to develop bioassays proved advantageous. He later commented: 'I felt it was the way forward because you learn much more about the mode of actions ... If you want [to] go *in vivo* ... it is very good for clinical relevance but if you want to find out how something works you are better off *in vitro* because it's a much simpler system. We developed a little assay based on vas deferens from the mouse which as it happens turned out to be stuffed full of cannabinoid receptors ... [It] turned out to be very sensitive to cannabinoids.'[38]

By the early 1990s Pertwee had demonstrated that he was able to work on mouse vas deferens using only tiny amounts of material. He presented some of the initial vas deferens data at a cannabinoid meeting in Palm Beach, Florida, in 1991, and this led to collaboration with Mechoulam. Here luck played a role. Mechoulam and Devane sent Pertwee some impure material, and Pertwee was able to discover that it paralleled THC in activity. On sending the pure substance, though, it was found to be inactive. This confusion was later cleared up when it was discovered that the pure material had oxidized and thus disrupted the experiment, whereas the impure material contained an antioxidant and was still effective for Pertwee.[39] As a result, using the mouse vas deferens, Pertwee (with Graeme Griffin) was able to provide the first evidence that this substance not only bound to cannabinoid receptors but also activated them. This strengthened the argument that anandamide was an endogenous cannabinoid that acted on the newly discovered receptors.[40] Pertwee explained how it was serendipitous that they used the vas deferens assays, as they had been working on other assays that could have provided a false trail: 'It was lucky we used this tissue, as gut chews up enzymes, so luckily, we used vas deferens. So, we were able to detect something.'[41]

The realization of the enormity of the impact of discovering the ECRS had a range of broader implications. The excitement led to a re-emergence of funding for the cannabis research field, and Pertwee has described how a flow of research funding emerged.[42] The new tranche of funding brought in new researchers. Pertwee received Wellcome Trust funding in the 1990s on a re-entry scheme, providing him with two new members of staff. An MRC cooperative scheme provided additional funding. The discoveries also led to the reinvigoration of the cannabis network and the establishment of international cannabinoid societies to advance the course of cannabis research. This in turn led to integration with several other scientific disciplines other than pharmacology and psychology. For instance, immunologists such as Dr Klein, professor of medical microbiology and immunology at the University of South Florida, were working in a new field of psychoneuroimmununology and finding areas of interest in research on cannabis.

After the discovery of the ECRS, new dedicated international societies and symposia that were much more open to new researchers were initiated. The International Cannabinoid Research Society met annually to exchange findings and to facilitate collaborations between scientists as well as with the pharmaceutical industry. Furthermore, a German clinician set up a specific society for research into medical applications: the International Association for Cannabis Medicine.[43] Dr Vincenzo di Marzio, a researcher on endocannabinoids in Italy, has explained its importance for CBMs: 'Some people view this issue as possibly separate from the remedicalization of cannabis but in fact we were getting many hints from knowing how the endocannabinoids are made and how they are regulated and how to use the plant cannabinoids.'[44] These scientific networks consolidated the field.

These developments provided cannabis therapeutics with a more acceptable face, because they explained the mechanism behind anecdotal reports of cannabis's benefits and the action of new cannabis-based drugs like nabilone. One reason the discoveries had such an impact on therapeutics was because the system impacted so many aspects of the body. Mechoulam described the excitement around the discovery: 'There is almost no major physical activity in which this system is not involved … It provided the basis for a huge amount of work.'[45]

In later decades the discovery of the ECRS led to new research, especially on the modulation of pain, neurodegenerative disease, and anti-inflammatory action. Other novel research areas included immunity, leading to research on how the ECRS might help prevent reoccurring tumour growth; treatment for post-traumatic stress disorder, where it appeared that it might play a role in emotions and memory function; use as an anti-inflammatory agent; for the treatment of schizophrenia; and for the treatment of some cardiovascular diseases. Alternatively, when the endogenous cannabinoid system malfunctioned, it appeared that it could lead to obesity, fertility problems, and stroke. The possibility emerged of manipulating the system to alleviate these disorders: a possibility that was of great interest to industry.

It was also important because the ECRS appeared to offer a way of avoiding one of the major hindrances to the use of cannabis as a medicine, and one that had previously frightened off industry: the psychoactive properties of the drug. Iverson has explained its significance: 'Using THC, or synthetic or cannabis extract, was always limiting ... a narrow window between desired result and intoxication. THC would also go everywhere in the brain whereas the endocannabinoid system could be much more specific. The discovery of the endocannabinoid system provided the potential for eliminating the intoxication element.'[46]

That the CB_2 receptor was located outside of the brain was of great interest to pharmaceutical companies because of the possibility of achieving pain relief without the 'high'. Other work by Pertwee's group in Aberdeen led to the discovery of the allosteric site on the receptor.[47] Pertwee described this as acting rather like a volume control, allowing the activity of the receptor to be turned up or down.[48] A new research aim was to develop drugs to enhance the activity of the receptor. The discovery of the ECRS meant that pharmaceutical companies finally developed a sustained interest, because they could look for either agonist or antagonist (receptor blocking) drugs that would affect the ECRS. Iverson later explained the importance to medicine: 'After all most of the drugs on the market ... the new drugs over the last twenty years ... are based on being agonist or antagonist of receptors of endogenous compounds like dopamine and so on.'[49]

The goal was to take this new understanding from the laboratory and make it feasible for use in the clinic, but the time lag between discovery and patients receiving the benefits could be considerable. Iverson later commented: 'Thirty years from lab discovery to useful medicine ... takes many decades. So, research is at an interesting stage. Modern neuroscience development will take a long time to reach maturity.'[50]

The discovery of the mode of action of cannabis finally caught the serious interest of pharmaceutical companies on two grounds. Either they could produce a medicine directly based on cannabis, or they could move away from cannabis-based drugs and towards endogenous cannabinoids, which would block (antagonists), mimic (agonists), or augment (agonists) the ECRS. This attracted Avensis, a leading pharmaceutical company, due to potential applications for treating obesity, which was potentially a high money-earning application. The company developed synthetic antagonists and agonists such as SR141716A, known as rimonabant and marketed as Acomplia. Sanofi has argued that obesity became a major public health concern, and one with potential mass market appeal for industry. Rimonabant was not without problems, because it became linked to depression, and it was withdrawn from the market. But the discovery of the ECRS had brought a novel dimension to research, as this understanding allowed some studies to move away from CBMs like the synthetic THC-based Marinol. It opened up a whole new arena and would lead to drugs that were well outside the remit of the MDA or the international drugs control conventions.[51] However, the drugs that were developed from this new understanding were still a long way off reaching the clinic, and over the next decade many studies remained focused on the plant-based or synthetic cannabinoids.

It was possible that the stigma around cannabis had created a glass ceiling for research and was permeating even these new approaches. Di Marzio has commented on how the stigma was difficult to dispel: 'There has always been this kind of preconceived idea that those working in cannabinoids were doing something wrong ... You can get an idea ... how still the stigma is acting. There has been now – it's almost 15 years, it's 18 years, 19 years – since the discovery of the CB_2 receptor, and there have been several CB_2 synthetic, CB_2 selective agonists for this receptor which are totally devoid of any psychoactivity so they could easily bypass all the problems of the psychotropic activity of cannabis and still we know very little about this.'[52] Nevertheless, by 1990 there was a change in attitudes towards cannabis-based drugs.

Cannabis derivatives like dronabinol were viewed more leniently in some quarters. At the request of the CND, the WHO reviewed dronabinol again in 1989 and argued for it to be downgraded, as it acknowledged that dronabinol's medical properties were greater than for the substances classified alongside it: 'It is nevertheless obvious in the assessment of the Committee that dronabinol has therapeutic usefulness that is definitely greater than that of the other substances in Schedule I which have very limited if any therapeutic usefulness and that it is comparable to that of a number of drugs in Schedule II.'[53] Furthermore, the WHO did not rate highly dronabinol's ability to adversely affect cannabis misuse as cannabis use was already widespread: 'Since cannabis is controlled under the Single Convention ... changes in the scheduling of dronabinol ... would not entail any change to the control status of cannabis. Nevertheless, there might be a concern about the possibility that the official recognition of therapeutic usefulness of dronabinol might encourage the medicinal use of cannabis and thus its abuse. However, cannabis is already the most widely abused illicit drug in the world ... It is unlikely that such recognition would make a significant difference.'

In 1991 the CND recommended rescheduling dronabinol from Schedule I to Schedule II.[54] This still left it a tightly controlled drug, and pressure built later for further downgrading. In the United Kingdom it was moved to Schedule II of the MDA regulations, placing it alongside morphine, though it remained an unlicensed drug and it had to be imported for prescription on a named-patient basis. This left the legal responsibly with the doctor. In 2002 the WHO recommended its downgrading to Schedule IV of the UN Convention on Psychotropic Substances, the lowest Schedule: 'The abuse liability for dronabinol is expected to remain very low so long as cannabis continues to be readily available ... The committee considered that dronabinol should be rescheduled to Schedule IV of the 1971 Convention on Psychotropic Substances, and to avoid placing stereochemical variants of the same substance under different control systems the committee recommended that all stereochemical variants of delta-9-THC be moved to Schedule IV of the 1971 Convention.'[55]

The stigma attached to cannabis still operated, and the recommendation was withdrawn on the advice of the UNODC. In 2006 the WHO recommended instead that it be transferred to Schedule III as a compromise, but it faced strong opposition.[56] Nevertheless, the endocannabinoids, especially anandamide, became major areas of study, though none by this stage had reached the clinic due to a lack of toxicity data. In the clinic the focus remained on THC, CBD, and CBN.

THE EMERGENCE OF GW PHARMACEUTICALS:
CANNABIS-BASED MEDICINE EXTRACTS, 1998–2007

Another avenue for research was the reinvestigation of herbal cannabis, and this route took off in the United Kingdom with the development of a small biotechnology company that was based on the development of extracts from the cannabis plant. Nineteen ninety-eight marked a new era in the development of CBMs with the establishment of GW Pharmaceuticals in the United Kingdom by the scientist entrepreneur Dr Geoffrey Guy and Brian Whittle. GW gained the first Home Office licence to cultivate, possess, and supply cannabis for research. Cultivation began in August 1998, from which GW produced Sativex, an oral-metered spray of a standardized extract from cloned cannabis plants. This marked a departure from the synthetic THC-based medicines of the 1970s and 1980s. Sativex was based on the use of extracts, and it contained THC and CBD in a 50/50 mixture.[57] The creation and development of GW marked a watershed in the process of the medical use of cannabis, reflecting changes in the state of the pharmaceutical industry; relationships between industry, government, academia, and patients; and developments in drug technology and clinical trial methodology.

But why did 1998 see the entry and sustained development of a pharmaceutical company in the United Kingdom that was specifically based on cannabis? Guy has discussed the increased interest from both researchers and patients in whole-plant-based medicines that happened around this time: 'The decision by the UK government to grant GW Pharmaceuticals the licence necessary to initiate cultivation and devise extraction procedures equal to the task of producing standardised plant extracts of proven content and stability was both timely and judicious coinciding as it did with a renewed interest generally in plant-based medicines. It is also relevant that many researchers and patients have concluded that the whole plant is more effective as medicine than THC alone especially in the form of synthetic analogues.'[58]

Cannabis medicines in the nineteenth century had been based on herbal cannabis, usually in the form of a tincture, but these medicines, in an era focused on the active principles of plants, had fallen by the wayside. With the discovery of cannabis's active principle, THC, interest in cannabis had produced pills such as nabilone (Cesamet) based on one synthetic active principle of cannabis. GW was

based on a different concept, whereby it aimed to capture something more akin to the whole plant. This alternative approach took
place within the context of changes in pharmacy and developments
in phytomedicine.

For most of our history, plants have been the main providers of
medical drugs, and even when it was pushed to the sidelines there
was a fluctuating but continuous interest in plant-based medicine.[59]
Plant medicine was important early on: quinine and pyrethrum
were the lynchpins for the treatment and control of malaria, for example. At the very time when synthetics were at their height, and
medicinal plants were marginalized in the West, some uncertainty
existed over the former's long-term sustainability, and hence there
remained a residual level of interest in plant-based medicine.[60] By
the 1970s, the continuing threat of old diseases such as malaria,
the increasing focus on diseases like cancer, and newly emerging
diseases such as AIDS, combined with increasing drug resistance,
provided impetus to find alternatives: this included the reinvestigation of plants and a greater interest in synergistic effects. Equally,
in the wider community, concerns over biomedicine, and a vague
unease that life had become too divorced from nature, increased
support for 'alternative' medicine. In addition, countries such as
Brazil and China had retained an ongoing and important relationship with traditional plant medicine.

While reservations remained over the potential value and usefulness of plants, increased acceptance of plant medicine emerged
among the public, in scientific circles, and in regulatory authorities.
Mead has discussed the role of patient advocacy in softening regulatory authority attitudes towards botanical medicines: 'The natural
foods movement reinforced by patient advocacy and empowerment
has also given new vigour to the interest in botanical medicine and
dietary supplements. Renewed support for botanical and other natural products has been accompanied by an increased distrust of
the pharmaceutical industry and its new chemical entities ... Regulatory authorities have become more receptive to the concept of
botanical medicines.'[61]

Despite, according to the WHO, cannabis having lost its medical
utility by the 1950s, and cannabis tincture having been removed in
the United Kingdom by 1973, in some spheres there was a renais-
sance in the appreciation of plant-based medicine. The National
Cancer Institute in the United States reflected this attitude. Its

screening programme for products that might be helpful in the fight against cancer initially excluded plants, but by the 1960s the Institute deemed it advisable to incorporate them. Two major developments – one in oncology around Taxol for cancer chemotherapy, and another around *A. annua* for the treatment and prevention of malaria – encouraged the revival of interest in plant-based medicines and insecticides.[62]

Primary health care accorded traditional medicine, in which plant lore was critical, a higher place within health policy. The Alma-Ata Declaration of 1978 and the WHO 'Health for All' report (1981) brought about a reassessment of approaches to public health, and one aspect of these changes was the increased consideration given to traditional medicine. The WHO report stated: 'The primary health care approach ... also emphasizes the need to make maximum use of all available resources. This is why the International Conference on Primary Health Care, in Alma-Ata in 1978, recommended that governments give high priority to the utilization of traditional medicine and the incorporation of proven traditional remedies into national drug policies and regulations.'[63]

The renewed focus on traditional medicine meant that plant-based medicines saw something of a revival from the 1980s onwards. In 1988 the International Union for Conservation of Nature (IUCN) and the WHO collaborated to produce guidelines on medicinal plant conservation,[64] and significantly the WHO published 'Traditional Medicine and Medicinal Plants': 'The recent decision to make the traditional medicine programme part of the global programme concerned with drug management and policies recognizes the importance of plants as sources of products of medicinal value, and the need for an adequate technological infrastructure to realize the potential.'[65]

Plants, however, provided a set of problems for industry. The problems highlighted in recent histories of plant-based medicines such as Taxol and *A. annua* can also be seen in the history of cannabis. Issues over supply, the isolation of active principles, standardization, and patents combined to create a challenging set of factors that made pharmaceutical companies reluctant to invest. Goodman and Walsh's work on the history of Taxol illustrates this: 'Few companies are capable of extracting and purifying large quantities of Taxol. Scaling up required capital investment and given the general lack of interest both in natural product medicine and anti-cancer agents among pharmaceutical manufacturers, there was probably a reluctance to invest.'[66]

Guy has elaborated on some of these issues and the niche they provided for the creation of GW:

> It was anticipated that one of the larger pharmaceutical companies would pick up the baton and use its vast drug development machinery to bring the project to fruition. Two major problems emerged. First, established 'big pharma' is not comfortable generally with development of phytomedicines from starting materials that have a history of abuse ... It prefers an established drug development paradigm in which research is carried out to define the 'active constituent'. This is thought to maximize intellectual property rights ... Second, in an environment where opinion is divided on the ethics of developing a cannabis-based product the boards of major companies probably reflect this dichotomy.[67]

Established pharmaceutical companies, who were uneasy about working with cannabis, left a space in the medical marketplace. The emergence of the biotechnology industry provided a new means to fill the space.

The biotechnology industry, which is the industrial application of biological processes, took off after the discoveries around DNA in the 1970s in the United States, and it developed in the United Kingdom after the 1980s.[68] As research and development and the cost of bringing drugs to market spiralled, acquisitions and mergers were commonplace in the pharmaceutical industry in the 1990s. National governments, especially in Britain and Germany, recognized the potential of biotechnology and encouraged its development via government initiatives and finance. New small companies emerged, focusing on niche markets, impacting the structure of industry. Quirke has explained the impact of the changed environment: 'It has brought back the inventor, in the person of the scientist-entrepreneur heading start-up companies. It has pushed big pharma into strategic alliances with start-up companies and academics and has led to the growth of what has been termed the bioscience industry.'[69]

The new structures encouraged innovation, and biotechnology firms contributed new therapies.[70] It was in this context that an entrepreneur in the biotechnology industry could start up a company to fill a niche area with a plant-derived CBM.

Geoffrey Guy, a physician with a degree in pharmacology from the University of London and one of the founders of GW Pharmaceuticals, had been involved in the pharmaceutical development of chemical entities, biotechnology products, and drug-delivery systems. He has summed up why he was the man to do the job: 'There was no-one else who was interested in making, or thought it was remotely possible to make, a medicine out of cannabis ... I'd had twenty years in narcotic analgesics, drug delivery, plant medicines and had just retired two days earlier ... and had the time to think.'[71]

Guy had had a long-term interest in plant-based medicines and had founded Phytopharm PLC in 1990, which developed novel products from medicinal plants and which he floated in 1996. He has explained the regulatory difficulties that had emerged when working on plant-based medicines in an era that concentrated on single chemical entities: 'Since the war, and certainly since the 1960s and the Dunlop Report and afterwards, the medicines regulation pertained to single chemical entities. The prospect of developing a medicine, which contains something like 420 chemicals in the modern regulatory environment, was considered in the late 1980s–mid-1990s to be pretty nigh impossible.'[72]

He became interested in building on his experience of plant-based medicine and aimed to 'bottle the essence of cannabis'. This meant the use of more than one active ingredient of cannabis and the use of herbal synergism. Scientists had been arguing since 1900 over the relative value of the alkaloids in cinchona and the possible benefits of drug combinations. In the 1990s, Kirby, a member of the department of medical parasitology at the London School of Hygiene and Tropical Medicine, developed the argument that a herbal mixture was more effective than the use of a single active principle. Combination drug therapy, for instance, had been developed in the AIDS field.[73] The decision of GW to use a mixture of extracts from cannabis in order to capture its essence was in stark contrast to earlier industry moves. In following this route, GW set out to produce something closer to the plant-based product smoked by many patients.

The establishment of GW reflected the relationship between industry and science. Historians such as Oudshoorn have shown how the demarcation between industry and universities has become increasingly blurred since the early twentieth century.[74] Lowy has demonstrated how the pharmaceutical industry has developed through close association with academic researchers.[75] In the case of cannabis, knowledge exchange between industry and academia proved crucial, and active attempts to integrate the two worlds were made from the 1990s onwards. International networking and the development of symposia facilitated an exchange of ideas and, importantly, opened a window to industry. The formation of societies such as the International Cannabinoid Research Society brought companies into contact with academics.[76] Guy has expanded on how one of these conferences restimulated his interest in the subject:

> I went to a conference in London … and … I thought:
> 'Ho hum, this is interesting. I thought it was … very taboo.'
> … And there was the MCA … the Home Office, some very
> eminent scientists … patients and patient groups, and a
> little smattering of pharmaceutical people … keeping their
> heads way, way down, because they didn't want to be seen
> at a cannabis conference. The question arose: if research
> is to be done on cannabis, how do you standardize it? …
> I stood up, spoke from the floor … and said that it could
> be done as long as you got the agreement from the Home
> Office, from the MCA.[77]

As with many new biotechnology firms, GW capitalized on networks between industry and academia. The company created an internal Cannabinoid Research Institute designed to provide links between commercial enterprise and academia. It was directed by Philip Robson, a consultant psychiatrist from the University of Oxford, who had provided a review on the therapeutic use of cannabis for the Department of Health in 1996. GW Pharmaceuticals began collaborations with many of the major players, including Professor Roger Pertwee, who was engaged as director of pharmacology at the company. Pertwee remained based at Aberdeen University but received funding from GW Pharmaceuticals to carry out work on plant cannabinoids. Further links were developed with Mechoulam and di Marzio. These networks between science and industry allowed both to benefit from the other's expertise.

Starting up such a firm involved a high level of risk, and nowhere more so than in the case of cannabis, where fears over safeguarding intellectual property rights and overcoming difficulties related to international drug controls made most other people steer well clear. Robson has described some of the risks involved: 'At that time in every country it was completely illegal. So in order for the thing to get off the ground you've got to convince the Home Office to give you a special licence which no one had done. Guy risked money before the Home Office came round to his repeated requests. There was no guarantee this would happen ... He took the risk and put his own money up.'[78]

The legal situation surrounding cannabis was still a major issue. But pressure from medicinal-user activists provided incentives for policymakers to define the boundary between therapeutic cannabis and recreational cannabis, a distinction which the synthetic drugs like nabilone had failed to achieve. Guy commented that 'the government was very concerned about the MS patients being pushed up Whitehall as a campaign to have cannabis legalized.'[79] So, by 1997 industry and policy interests were beginning to move in a similar direction.

Cannabis was a highly unusual substance in that it muddied the boundary between a medical and a recreational drug and was a drug that already existed in herbal form for both uses, in the public domain. This scenario provided ammunition to both those in favour of medicalizing cannabis and those determined to prohibit it. Robson has expounded on the difference between bringing any new drug to market and bringing cannabis to market, as well as the potential benefits of doing so from a legal and a public health viewpoint:

> The stuff is already out there in a totally unregulated
> way, manufactured by criminals whose quality control
> interests are not really at the forefront of their priorities.
> It's a paradox because if cannabis-based medicine was
> pharmaceutically produced and regulated a proportion
> of people currently running a risk by smoking illegal
> cannabis of uncertain strength and purity would switch to
> the pharmaceutical product and therefore even if there
> was an inherent risk in cannabis-based medicine you
> would be teasing out all the additional risk of smoking an
> unstandardized, possibly adulterated drug. Also, its illegal
> nature... the simple fact they could be arrested, even if
> not harmed directly by the medicine. It's a total mystery

to me why regulators wouldn't factor that into their calculations.[80]

Guy had approached government previously but had been advised to maintain his interest in opiate-based medicines research. He recalled: 'In the early 1990s we'd approached the Home Office and said: "I'd be interested in looking at cannabis," because, as you know, we'd dealt with the opium plant with opiates. We got a bit of a flea in our ear actually: the Home Office in the early 1990s said "No, you're going to stick with your opiates." And, like any other pharmaceutical company or chairman, I thought that we had other fish to fry, and so we did.'[81]

However, as is discussed in chapter 7, a major report by the House of Lords on therapeutic cannabis pressed for industry involvement.[82] As far as Robson was concerned, the House of Lords report conferred credibility and was vital for giving confidence to the industry: 'I don't think there would have been a GW if there hadn't been a House of Lords.'[83] The significance for industry was that the report opened the way for clinical trials and the potential licensing of a CBM.

The need to split medical arguments from calls for legalization provided encouragement. Confidence was boosted when David Blunkett, the Home Secretary, appeared supportive when he stated the following: 'Should, as I believe … this programme be proved to be successful I will recommend to the Medicines Control Agency that they should go ahead with authorising its medical use.'[84] Edwards has described the pressure for additional pain medicines: 'So, I think the official mind-set would have been … that one should be very willing to determine the therapeutic value of THC, even if it were dangerous because we knew we needed better drugs for pain relief. The pain specialists really made us feel a bit ashamed if we thought that morphine and heroin were enough – they weren't. We needed better drugs.'[85]

Guy has described how the government position did not deviate from its overall aim: to facilitate research and to oversee the development of a pharmaceutical-grade product, in order to eliminate the argument for legalization on medical grounds. He says:

If a product could be approved by the MCA as an approved
medicine then the government would move to reschedule
that product – not cannabis – not the plant, not the
raw material, but that finished product – they would

reschedule it to an appropriate schedule so that it could
be used as a medicine. Therefore it was the government's
position before I even got involved with them because
their concern was, if there is a medicine here, you have
to separate it from the advocacy debate. That's what was
done, very, very straightforward and very quickly then
… The government was entirely consistent all the way
through, and we got an enormous amount of support
from the Home Office, even directly from Cabinet Office
in the early days to ensure that this programme would run
ahead smoothly.[86]

Once government had determined that this was the way forward,
they needed to attract industry interest. Guy has described how the
doors were opened for his company at a witness seminar held in 2009:

Paul Boateng opened the meeting and said, 'Her Majesty's
Government has no will to reschedule cannabis', at which
point everybody's eyes went to the ceiling. 'However,' he
said, 'we'd like the research to be done.' At which point
most people thought: 'Well, this is bizarre.' But he did
suggest that if one wanted to do the research, one should
approach the Home Office Drugs Inspectorate [HODI].
Having worked in one of the most highly regulated
environments the previous 20 years with opiates and with a
range of materials like that, when a Minister says, 'Go and
see my officials', that's what we did.[87]

Guy met with the HODI and was surprised by their rapid response:
'We presented … to the Home Office in the January 1998, and I
nearly forgot about it again, because I thought it would be buried
in there for two or three years. About four weeks later I received a
phone call from the Chief Inspector of the Home Office, [who] in-
dividually is probably more responsible than anybody else in this
room for the progress of our programme, and that's Mr Alan Macfarlane. He rang me up and said, "We'll do this. We don't know how
we're going to do this: could you put a proposal in?"'[88]

The Home Office granted GW a licence to grow cannabis in June
1998, as well as a clinical trial exemption certificate to conduct
clinical studies with CBMEs for numerous applications. With these

permissions in place, GW was sufficiently confident to start the first large-scale, legal, and commercial enterprise that would produce cannabis for medicine in the United Kingdom.

LEARNING TO GROW CANNABIS: STANDARDIZATION, SECURITY, AND PATENTS

Uniformity is king. Everything we do strives to produce batch after batch of plant material which is almost the same as the one before.[89]

GW solved the problem of supply that had plagued cannabis research by turning to vertical integration, producing both the raw material and the finished product. The main issue for GW was the need to standardize the raw material. In describing his work, Dr David Potter, the chief botanist at GW Pharmaceuticals, highlighted the importance of standardization.[90] Standardization was another reason why industry steered clear of plants. These were products where external and uncontrolled forces, e.g. climate, could make it difficult to achieve the standardization of relative levels of active ingredients, and therefore of the dose. Goodman described the problem for Taxol: 'Yield and weather conditions were two elements that could not be controlled and had a considerable impact on the planning of clinical trials.'[91] For GW one of the main aims became the production of pharmaceutical-grade cannabis through growing genetically identical material in optimum uniform conditions.

Security issues also needed to be resolved. The placement of cannabis within the drug control mechanisms meant that special requirements for the site had to be met. A site was found where a security system was already in place, and which also provided a well-equipped research glasshouse and half an acre of space. As well as his botanical knowledge, Potter also brought with him useful police contacts built up in his earlier career in pesticides, and this facilitated the development of good working relationships with the police and the Home Office. Providing the necessary security was feasible but expensive, and later the site was split to spread risk.

The Home Office was particularly nervous about any diversion of plant material, so traceability was critical. Any failure to trace a particular plant and to tally numbers on any given day during a regular visit by the Home Office resulted in nerve-racking moments.

Potter described the paperwork as phenomenal.[92] Each plant had a unique number, and any movement, harvesting, or destruction had to be logged. Failure to meet Home Office requirements could have resulted in the removal of the licence and the failure of the project. Over time the relationship with the Home Office and the police settled down, and a spin-off was that the company could provide the police and the Home Office with specialist training courses on cannabis.

In seeking a standardized product, botanical knowledge was an essential prerequisite. Potter had seventeen years of experience working for Shell on pesticides, and he was experienced in the process of registering novel compounds. Suitable plant material had to be sourced, and as this was the first time that cannabis had been grown commercially on this scale in the United Kingdom, knowledge about growing the plants had to be acquired. This is where a company called HortaPharm BV in the Netherlands proved useful.

Staffed by expatriate Americans who had been banned from working in the United States, they had foreseen a time when there would be a demand for a range of cannabinoids, not just those producing high levels of THC. HortaPharm had combed the world for different seeds and had created a seed bank from which they had cross-bred plants in order to produce varieties with high degrees of cannabinoids, such as CBD. GW bought the rights to HortaPharm's collection and capitalized on the firm's intellectual knowledge.

International regulations forbade the movement of plants from the Netherlands to the United Kingdom, and as there was no system for granting Home Office permits for plants, only seeds could be transported, which did not fall under international regulation. HortaPharm was able to return to their parent plants to produce seeds that would produce similar progeny. These yielded eight packets of seeds of the most promising lines, which contained pure lines of CBD and THC. Eventually, as GW established itself, it was able to obtain licences for HortaPharm's collection of plants, which was transported to the United Kingdom, providing a resource which could be dipped into when necessary.

On 24 August 1998 the eight varieties produced by HortaPharm were planted, and ten days later they yielded the first 2,000 seedlings. HortaPharm provided the know-how to take the cuttings, and GW developed the process. Plants with the highest cannabinoid concentration and purity were identified: ten genotypes were selected and five were recommended for trial. These five chemovars (chemical varieties) were selected for commercial cultivation. Thus, GW had successfully bred the raw material and was therefore in a position to mass-produce standardized, or rather genetically identical, plant material, cloned from the original mother-plants raised by HortaPharm in 1984.

GW had to be able to control the growing environment. Potter has expanded on the need for standardization in phytomedicine: 'Medicinal cannabis must be of consistent quality. In striving to produce cannabinoids of uniform high quality commercially, the pharmaceutical company needs to ensure that plant material with the most appropriate genetics is selected for the propagation process ... The correct environment has to be found in which this material can be propagated, carefully harvested and stabilised by prompt drying.'[93]

When growing the plants to maturity, GW fine-tuned information from HortaPharm and incorporated the knowledge gleaned from illegal growers. The varieties that were resistant to pests, plant density, the growing medium, and humidity levels were all factors to be ascertained and controlled. Optimum conditions were found through a combination of trial and error and serendipitous discovery. One major issue was that the company was growing plants north of the equator, whereas cannabis that produces a higher concentration of active ingredients does not grow naturally in light levels found in the United Kingdom. Similarly, the plants were unable to produce enough harvests per year to keep pace with commercial mass production. Lighting in the greenhouse had to be supplemented to achieve standardized light levels and therefore standardized yields. The timing of harvesting was critical: one week early or late affected yields. Plants were cultivated in accordance with good agricultural practice methods from the European Medicines Evaluation Agency and in conjunction with the MCA, in order to produce a botanical drug substance.[94] Standardized cannabis plants were then ready for processing.

Intellectual property rights protection was essential for the company. Companies had tended to steer clear of plants in the past due to the difficulty of obtaining patents, and those that risked involvement faced debates over issues of biopiracy.[95] There were fears raised over the 'hijacking of an ancient and folk remedy' and 'the patenting of traditional knowledge'.[96] But standardization was a means of achieving property rights over the end product. GW was able to exploit this because it could certify a new variety as defined by the demonstration of distinctiveness, uniformity, and stability, therefore gaining European plant breeders' rights. This process would normally be carried out in the United Kingdom, but because of security issues plants could not be assessed in the United Kingdom and instead had to be exported to the Netherlands, incurring further difficulties over import and export licences, a process which caused some amusement at customs: 'Carrying cannabis to Holland?!'[97] Achieving standardization therefore provided an opportunity to obtain intellectual property rights, which was a necessity for making a high-risk investment worthwhile, as it allowed GW to license chemically and genetically characterized extracts of *Cannabis sativa* L.: CBD and CBN, protected as Tetranabinex and Nabidiolex, respectively.

Was all the effort worthwhile? After three years, GW was ready to test the product. Safety concerns over its impact meant that early tests on humans involved a ratio of one patient to thirteen doctors waiting to see what would happen. One patient became 'high' rapidly and described the medicine as powerful, like two joints of the best cannabis. Potter described the excitement: 'It told us we'd managed to capture the essence of cannabis in a bottle.'[98] While it was not the effect desired for a medicine, it proved that GW had achieved an action more closely related to that of herbal cannabis.

The decision by GW Pharmaceuticals to develop a new delivery system rather than staying with the oral administration method used for dronabinol (Marinol) and nabilone (Cesamet) leads to the question of how far technical change had helped to define a boundary shift from an illicit drug to a licit medicine. Producing oral cannabis medicines in the 1980s was important as a delineator of medical/non-medical boundaries, and it continued to be important especially in a climate that was increasingly anti-smoking. The spread of no-smoking zones to include hospitals, and also fears over lung damage, precluded the smoking route for acceptable evidence-based medicine.

However, oral medicines also had their detractors, and developments of alternative delivery methods have been important in the story of CBMs. It appeared that patients generally disliked the available oral cannabis-based tablets, as they had a long lag time and poor absorption. Nor was an oral route satisfactory for those suffering from nausea: this was one reason why tablets of dronabinol and nabilone were not frequently used. Intravenous and inhalation methods remained the quickest routes of absorption, but both had problems. Inhalation was initially proposed, but it presented technical problems.[99] Russo has shown how GW modernized the nineteenth-century technique of dissolving an extract in an ethanol base by utilizing supercritical CO_2 extraction. GW piloted propellant-powered aerosols, providing a fluid extract of a metered spray under the tongue or inside the cheek. This method allowed for reliable and rapid absorption, and it was a delivery method where patients themselves could self-titrate. Self-titration was important. As Notcutt recalled: 'I think that during the 1990s we also got used to the concept of patient-controlled analgesia after surgery.'[100] It put patients back in control of dosage.

The development of delivery methods has been historically important, as delivery methods and technological developments could provide intellectual property rights. This was an essential aspect of working with botanical products. GW developed specialist security technology that could be incorporated in all its drug-delivery systems, allowing the recording and the remote monitoring of patient usage to prevent any potential abuse of the company's CBMs. This technology enabled the industry to move medical cannabis further away from fears over misuse. By 2001 the company was ready to start clinical trials with Sativex.

CONCLUSION: PHYTOMEDICINE, THE
BIOTECHNOLOGY INDUSTRY, AND THE ROLE
OF THE INDIVIDUAL ENTREPRENEUR

Remedicalization was intimately linked with developments in the pharmaceutical industry. Over the period under study the pharmaceutical industry developed a greater interest in cannabis as a potential medicine. Initially, academic research had struggled without an industrial supply, but from the 1970s interactions between academia and industry boosted remedicalization and the development of CBMs. Nabilone and dronabinol set a precedent for the use of CBM and provided the cannabis therapeutics field with new legitimacy. However, the relative failure of these synthetic, single chemical entity drugs left the door open to patient pressure for access to cannabis and later forced a re-evaluation of herbal cannabis.

Pharmaceutical interest was re-stimulated when industry compounds contributed to new understandings of the mode of action of cannabis. This opened up two routes for industry involvement. Firstly, drugs were designed to manipulate the cannabinoid receptor system, which moved drugs away from cannabis itself. Secondly, industry involvement, stimulated by developments in phytopharmacy, moved research back in the direction of plant-based medical products and linked research more closely to the traditionally smoked herbal cannabis or the original herbal tincture of cannabis, whose mechanism of action had been revealed.

In the United Kingdom GW Pharmaceuticals, and its development of Sativex, spurred on the remedicalization of cannabis through the provision of a product that was more concurrent with developments in standardization, clinical trials, and drug regulation. The development of a new drug-delivery system, which was more effective and faster than the tablets used for the delivery of synthetic THC, and which steered clear of smoking, fitted within acceptable treatments but also took on board patient concerns.

If a licence was to be achieved for Sativex in the United Kingdom, it would be a remarkable development in the process of industrializing cannabis. Firstly, it would bring a cannabis-based drug back into the medical marketplace after the withdrawal of the extract. Secondly, although cannabis-based drugs like Marinol (dronabinol) had been on the market since the mid-1980s, these were based on synthetic THC, while Sativex consisted of extracts of cannabis, not synthetic derivatives. Thirdly, Sativex was based not on the use of one single active principle but on a combination of extracts of both THC and CBD, in an attempt to get closer to the 'whole plant'. Lastly, a new delivery system had the potential to provide the benefit of smoked cannabis without its negative connotations.

By 2001 GW was ready to start large-scale clinical trials by developing a portfolio of drugs and working on a range of applications beyond its starting point, which was a focus on treating MS. To bring its CBME product to market, Sativex had to pass successfully through the benchmark double-blind randomized clinical trial process and through the UK regulatory and licensing mechanisms. The following chapters consider the factors that contributed to the development of GW Pharmaceuticals and the process of bringing Sativex products through regulatory mechanisms: patient activism, expert committees, and clinical trials.

5

Forces of Necessity: Lay Advocacy and the Remedicalization of Cannabis, 1973–2001

Self-help and self-medication have always been important in the medical marketplace, and despite the increasing role of the NHS, health activism became important in the post-war period. This reflected a wider trend in activism that developed from the 1960s with the emergence of new organizations and charities. These organizations played an increasingly important role in society, e.g. Shelter helped the homeless and the World Wildlife Fund campaigned for conservation and wildlife. As Berridge has shown in relation to smoking, they were single-issue, media-aware, national organizations.[1] It was within this context that cannabis activism developed. Medical activism was one aspect of these early cannabis campaigns. Grassroots knowledge of drugs proved important for the growing relationship between the lay and professional spheres.

From the 1960s the focus of cannabis activism was on legalization for recreational purposes. Medical use was cited as one reason for this demand. In the United States individual patients campaigned for medical access to cannabis through the 1980s and 1990s, with patient associations joining the campaign later. These activists, however, distanced themselves from calls for legalization on recreational grounds. Medical access demands were then strengthened by the growing acceptance of cannabis as a treatment for the side effects of cancer chemotherapy. This was followed by the AIDS crisis of the 1980s, with the ensuing search for treatments adding pressure for access to cannabis and resulting in both the creation of new activist groups and cooperation with pre-existing cannabis activists. In the United States this activism changed policy, e.g. the setting up of compassionate access programmes in some states and the licensing of nabilone (Cesamet) and dronabinol (Marinol).

The impetus came from a different quarter in the United Kingdom. In the 1990s it was MS patients – both through patient associations that campaigned on cannabis as part of a wider remit and through activist groups that were set up as single-issue campaigning associations – who were demanding access to cannabis. This led to MS becoming the major stimulus for cannabis research.

Based on in-depth interviews and archival and documentary research, this chapter traces the role of lay advocacy in the remedicalization of cannabis, particularly in the United Kingdom, from the 1970s onwards. Through an in-depth analysis of the role of the MS Society and the Alliance for Cannabis Therapeutics (ACT), I argue that high-profile advocacy placed pressure on policymakers, leading to an outcome that changed attitudes in government towards clinical trials and that provided incentives for the pharmaceutical industry to become involved. The emphasis MS campaigners placed on respectability, married with their ability to forge cross-class alliances, was significant within this. The chapter also argues, following interviews with significant insiders, that advocacy was crucial in focusing the direction of research. The development of cannabis as a medicine has been brought about to a large extent by patient-led demand driving the scientific community, policy advisers, and industry to build on anecdotal and scientific knowledge.

MEDICAL NECESSITY 1975–91: GLAUCOMA, CANCER, AND AIDS

The cannabis activism initiated in the 1960s had focused on the liberalization of the legal framework surrounding cannabis. In some instances, activists extolled the medicinal properties of the plant, but their arguments were subsumed by the larger campaign to make recreational consumption more palatable to regulators. Perhaps the best-known pressure group in the United Kingdom was SOMA (Society of Mental Awareness), an organization founded by Stephen Abrams in 1967.[2] SOMA's network included a physician, a pharmacologist, and a research psychologist, but it drew on a wider set of supporters, ranging from Francis Crick, the co-discoverer of the structure of DNA, to The Beatles. SOMA attempted to influence policy through the media and through public opinion throughout the decade, with its most famous moment being the placement of an advertisement in *The Times* on 24 July 1967.[3] The advertisement was designed to influence the terms of reference of the Wootton Committee, which had been set up by the government to examine the case for law reform, and the advert was subsequently referenced in the introduction to the Wootton Report, published in 1968.[4] Such activism appeared to have little policy impact and the Wootton Report was rejected by the government.

These politicized campaigns for legalization failed due to a hostile policy environment. Arguments for medicinal cannabis were overwhelmed by fears over recreational use and limited proof of medical efficacy. Single-issue groups could be short-lived, and SOMA folded due to a lack of funds,[5] but successors followed: in 1978, for instance, the LCC was initiated to campaign for full legalization of the use and distribution of cannabis in the United Kingdom. The new LCC campaign demanded that cannabis products be made available for prescription by doctors without special requirements. Such arguments, however, were buried in the push for wider access to cannabis products in general, and for recreational consumption in particular. Separating the medical from the recreational proved to be an important next step.

Cannabis use for 'medical necessity' gained legal status in the United States; developments in the United States are worth reviewing because they influenced UK campaigners, who forged links with and built on the work of early US organizations. Emily Dufton, in particular, has explored the role of patient activism in the United States.[6] Robert Randall was instrumental in US medical cannabis patient activism. In 1972 Randall's glaucoma (a progressive disorder of the eye that destroys cells in the retina, degrades the optic nerve, and causes eventual blindness) forced him to search for alternative therapies. Conventional treatments at the time did not provide lasting effects, and surgery was ruled out. He was advised to plan for a life of disability. While smoking cannabis one night, though, Randall found that the blurred halos around the street lights were gone. He convinced himself and his partner, Alice O'Leary, that cannabis was the cause of this relief, and he began to grow the plant on his property to provide a regular supply. In August 1975 the house was raided, and Randall turned himself in to the police. A series of legal actions to establish the 'medical necessity' argument ensued. To this end, Randall successfully forged alliances in the scientific and medical communities, eventually proving that cannabis was an effective treatment for his condition, which saw him acquitted of the charges for possessing marijuana; he was also able to procure a legal supply of the drug.[7] When the FDA attempted to block this access, Randall brought a case against them in 1978 and won.

This second legal victory meant that the US government had to create a programme – the Compassionate Investigational New Drug (Compassionate IND) programme – to provide compassionate access to cannabis. Thereafter, the Compassionate IND programme supplied NIDA with cannabis for approximately thirty qualifying patients, a success that further encouraged patients to collaborate to push for legal access to cannabis for specific medical problems. Health activism then started developing on a larger scale. The campaigning morphed from small-scale cases to pressure for the reform of laws that denied access in the first place. In 1981, for example, Randall and O'Leary founded ACT. It was ACT that provided the template for an important activist organization in the United Kingdom in the 1990s. Overall, Randall's struggles were central to the process of separating the campaign for easier access to preparations of the plant for medical purposes from the wider movement to reform cannabis laws in the United States.

In the United Kingdom, meanwhile, the findings of the 1980 EGEC set up by the ACMD helped change attitudes towards cannabis. Composed of medical and scientific authorities, and chaired by J.D.P. Graham, a professor of pharmacology at Cardiff University, the ACMD downplayed the risks of cannabis. Attention, instead, began to focus on the possible benefits of cannabis substances, particularly for the treatment of side effects of cancer treatments.[8] Synthetic versions were produced, including nabilone (licensed in the United Kingdom in 1982) and Marinol (licensed in the United States in 1985). Cannabinoids were back on the agenda in medical science, but that did not necessarily include whole or herbal cannabis, such as the flowers, stems, or leaves, often either smoked or taken as a tea. Moreover, these scientific and regulatory developments were not sparked by patient activism but by patient need, from those in cancer care enduring chemotherapy.

HIV (human immunodeficiency virus)/AIDS activists and communities provided the next shift in the United States. Clinton Werner, a scholar of the American medical marijuana movement, has concluded that the 'experience of desperate AIDS patients using medical marijuana helped to change the national perceptions of the drugs from menace to medicine'.[9] An initial focus on the development of drugs to combat the infection drove the change. Much of the attention was, of course, focused on an antiretroviral medicine called AZT (azidothymidine). The side effects of AZT included headaches, nausea, and weight loss, however, which exacerbated the problems caused by AIDS. In self-help circles, herbal cannabis became popular, acting as an appetite stimulant and painkiller; but its usefulness was compromised by its illicit status.

Activism by AIDS patients was led by a well-organized gay rights movement that was experienced in political agitation on civil rights issues, and the ready-made network of cannabis campaign groups such as ACT proved invaluable for AIDS campaigners as well. Though cannabis-based drugs were available on the market, they were not available for applications other than as a palliative in specific cancer treatments. Herbal cannabis remained illegal. The Compassionate IND programme became a way for AIDS patients to gain access to an otherwise-illicit substance. The programme was a concession rather than a right, was limited to meeting patient demand, and had a tenuous place in federal law. Booth has argued that the fury at the closure of the Compassionate IND programme in 1992 led to further development of the grassroots movement to protect patients and also to the development of 'buyers clubs' for alternative and illicit remedies.[10] Members could join these clubs if they held a doctor's certificate stating that their condition would benefit from cannabis, but because the clubs remained illegal under federal law they were eventually closed down. The use of cannabis as an anti-nausea drug in relation to cancer chemotherapy had, however, established that cannabis-based substances could have a legitimate medical application – something that could be used as a precedent for AIDS treatment. Marinol was consequently made available on prescription for AIDS patients in 1992 in the United States. Patients already receiving herbal cannabis were allowed to continue, but those who were in the process of being placed in the compassionate programme were provided with Marinol; this enabled the US government to argue that the use of smoked herbal cannabis for medical purposes was obsolete.[11,12]

CANNABIS, MULTIPLE SCLEROSIS,
AND PATIENT PERSPECTIVES IN THE
UNITED KINGDOM, 1992–2007

In the United Kingdom it was MS – a progressive, degenerative disease impacting the brain and the spinal cord nerves – that impacted policy discussions about cannabis medicines. Orthodox therapies included baclofen (Kemstro) and diazepam (Valium) for the treatment of muscle spasms and spasticity, but their efficacy was limited and both had unpleasant side effects. MS patients faced a variety of symptoms for which there were no effective treatments, especially chronic and severe pain. In response, an educated and informed patient population started taking an increasingly active role in treatment options. In the 1990s different types of self-help groups became vocal in pressuring for research on cannabis to treat MS. These societies influenced the cannabis story, with each bringing a slightly different perspective and emphasis to advocacy on cannabis. Together they provided considerable pressure for research.

Some of these grassroots groups played an active role in the provision of information as well as of supply. THC4MS (Therapeutic Help from Cannabis for Multiple Sclerosis (UK)) aimed to supply information and later medicinal cannabis chocolate to MS sufferers. It was founded in 1998 following a debate about cannabis and MS on the Kilroy BBC television chat show, which enabled MS sufferers to meet and which provided a public platform. THC4MS relied on donations of raw cannabis from growers across the United Kingdom, and it then supplied the medicinal cannabis chocolate bar Biz Ivol to people with MS nationwide, becoming the subject of a BBC documentary in 2005. Early that same year, THC4MS was raided by the police, and three members were prosecuted for cannabis supply in 2004/5 and were handed sentences of nine months suspended for two years. Medical necessity was not deemed applicable in this case by the Court of Appeal in 2005 although it had previously been used successfully as a defence.

Other groups had a more profound effect on both policy debate and research. The MS Society, formed in 1953, was one of the earliest patient-activist groups. It had two major aims: to support patients with MS and to foster research into treatment. Cannabis became of interest in the 1990s, and the society argued that if cannabinoid-based medicine proved safe and effective in clinical trials then it ought to be made available to patients through the NHS. The society stipulated that research should be vigorously pursued and that cannabis must be judged equally to other treatments, namely, using the criteria that applied to the assessment of any proposal for a new drug therapy, with normal standards for quality, safety, and efficacy. The society funded a number of clinical trials. Its policy was not to recommend the use of herbal cannabis prior to clinical trials, though it did urge authorities to deal sympathetically with people who self-medicated. As the group told parliament: 'The MS society does not encourage people with MS to break the law. We do however understand why some people who face intolerable symptoms have chosen to make their own decisions about cannabis use ... Where the medical evidence warrants it, we hope that the police and the courts would deal with such people in an appropriate, compassionate fashion.'[13]

The MS Trust, set up by Jill Holt and Chris Jones in 1993, had a specific agenda to stimulate medical research into the condition. Both founders had personal experience of MS and had been involved with another group, Action and Research for MS (ARMS), an organization founded in 1974 to make applied research into MS a priority. ARMS disbanded in 1993, but Holt and Jones sought money to continue the research programme. They argued that applied research remained underfunded, that information for the newly diagnosed was inadequate, that the understanding of MS remained poor, and that NHS services were limited. A small charitable trust was established with two MS researchers. Clinicians described the trust as 'a breath of fresh air' in its willingness to provide resources, though their funding ability was limited.[14] While the MS Trust was more research-driven than the MS Society, cannabis was one of many options that it was willing to support.

ACT was set up in 1992 by Clare Hodges (also known as Dr Elizabeth Brice), an MS sufferer. ACT was based on the Alliance for Cannabis Therapeutics in the United States. In contrast to the MS Society and the MS Trust the UK ACT was created as a single-issue, single-activity self-help group for medicinal cannabis users, campaigning specifically for cannabis research and for direct access through the NHS. Hodges herself suffered from spasticity, loss of sensation, bladder problems, nausea, and diminished appetite. Nine years of orthodox medicine had provided limited sustained relief and many unpleasant side effects. After reading about cannabis in the *American Medical Journal*, she tried smoking cannabis and found that it alleviated some symptoms. She recalled her difficulties obtaining cannabis: '[As] a middle-class mother of two young children, I had a bit of [a] problem obtaining cannabis.' She eventually had help obtaining cannabis, and she found it beneficial: 'When I did try cannabis the physical relief was almost immediate ... I was comfortable with my body for the first time in years.'[15]

According to certain accounts, patient associations were largely a middle-class activity, and ACT/Hodges fitted this mould. Indeed, this perhaps worked to Hodges's advantage, by bringing a not so 'respectable' activity, cannabis consumption, into a 'respectable' setting.[16] She began to cultivate, smoke, and ingest herbal cannabis. With the introduction of nabilone she hoped to find a legal method of treatment, but instead she experienced unpleasant side effects, and it failed to produce the beneficial effects of herbal cannabis. With the licit cannabis-based drug having failed, from the patient's perspective, Hodges felt forced to revert to herbal cannabis. Her neurologist put her in touch with others who were self-medicating with herbal cannabis in 1992, and they decided to form a group to campaign for more research and to provide information to sufferers and to the public about medical cannabis issues. Hodges explained her motivation: 'I found out it was not just me ... so I raised awareness and let people know about it.'[17] The use of cannabis, however, posed problems from two points of view: the threat of prosecution and the lack of quality control, including unknown dosages.[18]

The UK ACT encouraged research into medical preparations of 'herbal or natural cannabis' and advocated for such therapies to be made available on a doctor's prescription while research was ongoing. As Hodges emphasized, this was a campaign not for legalization but rather for access to a medical drug via the NHS: 'We are not campaigning for the general legalization of cannabis. Indeed, even if cannabis were legalized we would still be campaigning, as we think seriously ill people should get their medication from their doctor and not have to provide it for themselves.' She went on: 'Similarly the objectives of ACT would not necessitate cannabis being legalized. Preparations of cannabis could be available for medical use whilst still being illegal as is the case for diamorphine/heroin.'[19] ACT argued that herbal cannabis had a long history in a medical setting and that it was safe and available. ACT went further than the MS

Society, arguing that patients needed immediate relief, not help at some undefined point in the future.

An important aspect of these three distinct patient associations was their ability to provide an interface between patients and researchers, drawing the lay and professional spheres closer together.[20] ACT developed close connections with scientists and the medical profession, and it was also able to provide laboratory scientists with access to patient perspectives. Hodges described the membership of ACT as a loose affiliation of patients (including those with spinal injuries and cancer), doctors, hospital consultants, and health workers. Its role was to help research to take place. For the scientists working on cannabis-based products, the association provided a willing pool of patients, many of whom were actively interested in the research. ACT also worked with the pharmacologist Professor Roger Pertwee, from Aberdeen University, on a project studying the perceived effects of smoked cannabis on patients with MS. ACT assisted by distributing questionnaires and by providing access to users. The links to the US ACT provided access to additional users as well.[21]

Similarly, interactions with clinicians were initiated. Hodges developed links with Dr William Notcutt, an anaesthetist who was carrying out work on nabilone for pain.[22] She was able to obtain nabilone on a named-patient basis rather than having to resort to the black market for herbal cannabis. This was rare. Here is Hodges explaining some of the difficulties involved in sourcing cannabis: '[Often] you can't get it from the doctor. There are only a handful of doctors that can do it. Others get it illegally from the black market but people are scared. They wrote to ACT, asking, "Where can we get it?" Most people just don't know where to get cannabis.'[23]

Patient–doctor relationships therefore provided a conduit for the patient perspective to reach the medical establishment. This was particularly important over the issue of the unsatisfactory nature of nabilone in comparison with herbal cannabis. Hodges described her attempt to move to the licit nabilone and to stay off illicit cannabis: 'I had just been prescribed nabilone … I took this for four nights but it made me confused and clumsy. I persevered hoping it might be a substitute, but it wasn't.'[24] It became clear to both patients and clinicians that further research was needed on other cannabis-based products, most notably herbal extracts, rather than a single chemical entity like nabilone.

Interactions between the MS Society and laboratory scientists partially contributed to a breakthrough in scientific knowledge about the role cannabis could play in MS treatment. Initially, the society had been cautious about cannabis research and had refused to fund trials in the early 1990s,[25] but by the late 1990s it was taking an interest, albeit cautiously. The society placed emphasis on 'respectability', which it believed it needed to maintain if it was to engage with an illicit substance. This was achieved by maintaining distance from legalization campaigns and from demands for access to cannabis prior to clinical trials. Dr Lorna Layward, an immunologist at the MS Society, explained some of the initial concerns: 'Legalise Cannabis,' she suggested, 'was the only strongly campaigning group at the time and we did not want to be involved in the issue of legalisation of an illegal substance.'[26]

Legalization campaigns were re-emerging in the 1990s,[27] and the MS Society was keen not to be associated with them. The society's initial remit did not cover the sponsorship of scientific research, mainly because of the antipathy of the medical establishment towards lay involvement.[28] The society had changed its position on funding basic science research by the late 1950s, but this led to disagreements over the allocation of scarce resources. The dilemma was that, on the one hand, the society called for patience in waiting for effective therapies, implying that they were imminent, but, on the other hand, it indicated that there was much research still to be carried out. Attention was directed towards understanding the disease, finding a cure, and eliminating the condition, rather than towards treatment and care. But with no cure in sight, the society was forced to take a greater interest in the alleviation of symptoms. Writers on the early history of the society have argued that it was the social background of the society's founding members and, in particular, its ties to neurology that made respectability especially important.[29] The society therefore placed great importance in its early days on remaining orthodox and on ignoring fringe medicine. Since it received a constant stream of letters on alternative treatments, the society saw MS as a disease that attracted a great deal of 'quackery'.

Yet, by the 1990s the society's membership, upset by the lack of effective treatments, started to look for alternatives. In 1994 a new chief executive, Peter Cardy, initiated a review of members' attitudes. Cardy asked Layward to investigate the potential of cannabis. She explained that her initial response to Cardy's request was one of caution: 'One of the early things the chief executive said to me was, "Is there anything in this cannabis story?", and I was incredibly reluctant ... My perception was that I did not want to get involved in legalisation but wanted to focus on scientific evidence.'[30]

Patient perspectives began to undercut such concerns. Layward, despite being reluctant, described the impact of the patient experience on her own attitudes when carrying out a survey on MS Society members and their reactions to cannabis: 'It is only when I started to speak to people with MS that I started to change my mind.'[31] Layward never forgot one patient's response: 'I remember distinctly a comment ... He/she said, "Bugger research, one puff and I can straighten my leg."'[32]

As these patient voices filtered through to the society's leadership, new approaches to cannabis were developed.[33] The discovery of the ECRS in the 1990s[34] provided some legitimacy to anecdotal accounts of the medicinal use of cannabis, but proof was needed of its value in specific applications, such as in MS. When investigating existing research on cannabis and MS, Layward made links with Pertwee, and also with Dr David Baker at the Institute of Neurology. Layward asked Baker to carry out systematic research into the effects of cannabis on MS, and she put him in touch with Pertwee.[35] Six to seven months were needed to develop equipment that would measure the effect; the project results showed that cannabis had a significant impact on tremors in mice – tremors that were similar to those experienced by humans with MS.[36] The experiment seemed to validate the patient experience. According to Layward: 'It showed for the first time objectively that cannabinoids could do what people with MS were telling us. What we had demonstrated was ... "one puff and I can straighten my leg".'[37] The results were published later on the front page of *Nature*, adding to emerging discussions about potential clinical trials.[38] Ultimately, the experiment had a worldwide impact and gained positive media reportage in the United Kingdom.[39] It was important because, as Baker recalled: 'It started to put biology behind the patient perspective.'[40]

The MS Society pushed for clinical trials to go ahead, as that was the only method of getting cannabis-based drugs to their members. ACT was keen on clinical trials, but it recognized that there would be a massive time lag between them taking place and the development of a medicine, so it preferred to pressure for immediate access to herbal cannabis: 'We want to see the problem addressed now as well as the research.' Hodges highlighted the need for faster solutions: 'You can do the two in conjunction.'[41] The MS Society, in contrast, justified its more cautious approach in the following way to the House of Lords in 1997: 'Any proposal for therapy has to conform to stringent medical standards ... Unless and until such trials are undertaken and a therapeutic benefit is demonstrated the MS Society would not support the prescription of cannabis for people with MS.'[42] The MS Society argued that, since MS was a long-term illness, any drug had to be effective and safe over the long term. In not advocating the immediate use of cannabis, and not advocating any change to the law surrounding cannabis, the group sought to maintain respectability and consequently to maintain its influence on policy and the medical environment.

Clinical trials therefore became of critical importance. As Layward put it: 'We had been aware of the anecdotal evidence of the benefits of cannabis for some time, but strongly believed that trials were essential to rigorously test the effectiveness of the drug and to develop safe and easy methods of use.'[43] The relationship between the MS Society and Anthony Moffat, the chief scientist at the RPS, was vital. Layward explained the convergence of interest in clinical trials by patient associations and professional bodies: 'We both had the same sort of viewpoint,' she contended. 'Not interested in legalisation ... What we were interested in [was] was there any medicinal use? That marriage ... that relationship was absolutely pivotal to making all of this happen.'[44] As it transpired, the MS Society joined forces with the RPS and the BMA in 1997, organizing an influential conference on clinical trials.[45] The society was wary, nervous of the press response and of the risk to its reputation; still, it seemed that it was an appropriate time for trials to proceed. According to Layward: 'We were pushing at a time when there was a lot of resistance but over the coming year the resistance fell away. There was the discovery of the cannabis receptor system, MS and HIV patients talking about cannabis in terms of making them feel better ... There was a clamouring from different groups of people and anaesthetists were interested in pain relief.'[46]

The symposium drew scientists, clinicians, patients, and, most importantly, funders together, focusing their attention on the provision of protocols for trials on MS and pain. It also attracted industry attention. ACT actively sought out the pharmaceutical industry to encourage the production of legal cannabis therapies. Several companies were contacted, but to no avail – cannabis therapies were seen as too controversial and not worth the investment. As Hodges recalled: 'One company ... took it quite a long way ... and told me in confidence that it was too controversial, the scheduling was too difficult, it just was not worth the investment.' However, Hodges was able to find someone who was interested but who had previously failed to obtain a licence, and she asked him to try again to obtain a Home Office licence: 'At the Royal Pharmaceutical Society last summer I met a man who is an ex-chairman of a pharmaceutical company and he had tried to get a Home Office licence and had preliminary discussions with them four years ago and he had been advised not to go ahead. Recently, I approached him and suggested that he have another go, and he tried again.'[47] Getting the pharmaceutical industry involved proved more difficult than expected.

The meetings organized by the Royal Pharmaceutical Society were significant though, because they enabled interactions with Geoffrey Guy, one of the founders of GW Pharmaceuticals, and with other stakeholders. For industry involvement to proceed, the approval of the Home Office was necessary. Patient groups were important here too, in placing pressure on the government. The MS Society and ACT sought to bring the patient perspective closer to policymakers. For example, they developed relationships with professional bodies, including the BMA. Influential reports on therapeutic cannabis, such as the BMA report that emerged in the 1990s, absorbed evidence given by ACT and the MS Society.[48] ACT was also especially effective at keeping the issue high on everyone's agenda through the media. Reflecting on applying pressure for change, Layward felt that patient activism was key: 'We couldn't get anywhere without those sorts of groups keeping the agenda high, ... [by] speaking to the press.'[49]

Press responses were largely positive towards medicinal cannabis use, and it was a popular human-interest topic.[50] 'Three hundred individuals wrote in about how much they had benefited from it,' Hodges noted. 'All grist to the mill, [it] wasn't just me. [It] doesn't take long for it to get around ... The press very much like running stories about it because most people in the press use it.'[51] This positive publicity highlighted the problems of prosecuting patients for trying to alleviate their symptoms, and it increased public support for their cause.

Links between activist groups and the policy community became increasingly important.[52] While the MS groups were not as closely

associated with a 'network of influence'[53] as some organizations
(such as Action on Smoking and Health (ASH), the anti-tobacco
group) were, they certainly sought to make a contribution to the
policy environment. ACT in particular began to lobby the government. It organized delegations to the Department of Health in 1994
and 1997 that included MPs, scientists, and clinicians. These stressed
the need for medicinal preparations of herbal cannabis to be made
available for research, and they also argued that prescriptions on a
named-patient basis should be provided.[54] Hodges courted sympathetic MPs such as Paul Flynn, and MS groups were involved in the
All-Party Parliamentary Group for MS.[55] This group, consisting of
MPs and peers with a specific interest in MS, was established in 1997
to promote the interests of people affected by the illness. This interaction at the heart of government enabled the patient associations
to draw attention to the MS issue and, within that, the need for clinical trials.

Patient groups also contributed to parliamentary expert committees. These committees will be discussed in depth in the next
chapter, but lay activists played a key role in their debates. The MS
Society and ACT were invited to present evidence to a House of Lords
committee on therapeutic cannabis during the late 1990s. Their evidence provided an opportunity to bring the patient perspective to
the House of Lords and to generate more public awareness of the issues. The organizations raised concerns over the lack of treatments,
the importance of clinical trials, and the form of the drug to be
trialled.[56] ACT also campaigned for access to herbal cannabis while
trials were being developed.

The MS Society, despite accepting many of the points made by
ACT, made it clear that they were not prepared to accept anecdotal
evidence nor to push for interim access to herbal cannabis in 1997.
They argued that clinical trial evidence for the efficacy of the new
drug beta interferon for MS symptoms was sufficient to justify prescription, and in the absence of comparative evidence for cannabis
the society could not support its use in clinical practice. They emphasized that it was 'essential that further research is taken', and
they steadfastly pressed the case for clinical trials. However, they
were concerned that clinical trials, because of the nature of the disease and the substance being tested, would pose complications. A
large section of their evidence was given over to the methodology
of potential clinical trials, predicting many of the problems that

would later emerge. In contrast to the initial policy of the society, they had begun to argue that disincentives for research were financial and attitudinal rather than legal, and that they were happy to fund research.[57]

By increasing the involvement of the interests and experiences of patients in deliberations, activists helped to shape the form of the debate in a way that had not occurred in the closed expert discussions of the 1970s. Differences of opinion existed on the importance of the House of Lords report in this process. While some, such as Philip Robson, the medical director at GW Pharmaceuticals, argued that it was critical to advance research,[58] Layward held the view that trials would have gone ahead without the report. 'We carried on,' she contended, and 'they came up with what we were doing anyway … It was because there was a groundswell. Without it, it still would have happened.'[59]

Geoffrey Guy, one of the founders of GW Pharmaceuticals, appeared hopeful when he gave evidence to the House of Lords committee in 1997: 'I think also that the new research here, which is very much patient-demand led, will be accompanied by funding for research programmes … The MS Society has already said they would support clinical trials … As yet there seems no prospect of any funding from government.'[60] When GW Pharmaceuticals found itself considering research into cannabis, it was in relation to MS precisely because activists had been so effective in establishing a link between the drug and the condition in the minds of the public and policymakers: 'MS is a major awareness group … So, at the beginning, a focus on MS was sensible,' recalled Robson.[61]

One area of contention was over the form of cannabis to be used: herbal cannabis or drugs derived from single, synthetic principles. Nabilone (a synthetic form of THC) had been licensed for treatment in cancer chemotherapy, but it could also be prescribed for MS patients. MS patients with experience of self-treating using herbal cannabis found that, as was the case previously with HIV/AIDS patients, the legal synthetic THC drugs appeared inferior in terms of their efficacy and their side effects. This experience was noted in the House of Lords report. Nabilone, according to the government document, was not an effective substitute for herbal cannabis: '[It] does not seem to be an effective substitute for cannabis used therapeutically … All those who have taken both nabilone and natural cannabis say that cannabis is more effective and easier to control.'[62]

ACT, for its part, campaigned for herbal cannabis.[63] The MS Society also argued that there might be many useful cannabinoids within cannabis or an interplay between cannabinoids. They pressured for a trial on herbal cannabis and another trial on specific cannabinoids, especially those that lacked a psychoactive element. In its presentation to the House of Lords committee, the society argued that the trials should have two different arms. [64] Furthermore, patient associations were involved in discussions over the mode of administration. In a survey, members of the MS Society expressed concern over the effect of smoking on their health, and the society doubted that any drug administered through this route would pass through the regulatory mechanisms. ACT offered a different perspective: 'With a disease so unpredictable, self-education seems more helpful than treatment with a regular dose of a fixed strength ... People gain from treating themselves ... Most people choose to smoke cannabis ... The advantages in taking cannabis via the lungs is that the effects are much quicker and therefore easier to regulate.'[65]

Lay activists were therefore critical in building pressure to hold clinical trials, and they also helped to shape their format. The role of MS associations in the open expert committees that changed the policy environment, enabling clinical trials to proceed in 2001, will be discussed in more detail in chapter 6; I explore the role of patient activism within the clinical trials and their outcomes in chapter 7. But patient activism largely tailed off after the turn of the millennium. The MS Society had other issues to campaign on, and its success in the development of clinical trials meant that the society's attention was diverted elsewhere. Hodges also provided a more prosaic explanation of why the lay advocates were less active in the subsequent decade: 'People with MS are weary and ill and haven't got the energy to campaign.'[66]

CONCLUSION

Lay knowledge and activism were critical to the remedicalization of cannabis in the United Kingdom from the 1990s. In the 1960s and the 1970s, pressure groups campaigned for the legalization of cannabis as part of a lifestyle choice. Within their arguments these pressure groups raised the issue of medical cannabis, but, since their main focus was on the politically contentious issue of legalization for recreational use, they had limited policy impact. As lay knowledge around cannabis's medical properties increased, advocacy based purely on medical arguments became prominent, especially in the United States in the late 1970s and the early 1980s. This resulted in the successful legal argument of medical necessity for the use of cannabis and the initial development of compassionate access. These campaigns, combined with developments in the scientific field, provided much greater legitimacy for cannabis's medical use.

The AIDS crisis then propelled the issue forward and achieved some changes with, for example, the expansion of compassionate access programmes, but it did not lead to lasting changes in policy. These arguments filtered through to the United Kingdom, where they stimulated the development of equivalent UK societies, but in the 1990s pressure emerged from a different quarter. MS patient associations were highly active in that decade, and they created a platform for the patient perspective to impact both the scientific and policy spheres. Though these societies had dissimilar approaches, their combined advocacy provided a respectable face for medicinal cannabis. Via lobbying efforts they kept the issue high on the agenda and encouraged the shift from anecdotal lay knowledge to the facilitation of evidence-based knowledge with the initiation and development of clinical trials. They brought herbal cannabis to the fore, demanding a product much more closely aligned with their own experience than the synthetic, single-active-principle-based substances that had previously made it to market.

In the United Kingdom the MS patient associations, particularly ACT (UK) and the MS Society, became examples of very active patient associations that interlinked with scientific and policy spheres. These societies had some differences of opinion and varying approaches, but their combined advocacy provided a respectable face for medicinal cannabis use. Patients had limited power in their own right: power lay in their knowledge and their ability to place pressure on other actors in the remedicalization process, especially after their experiences had been validated to some extent by the discovery of cannabis's mechanism of action. The patient associations were successful in presenting their case and became interlinked with, and inseparable from, the other main actors, including industry, the media, clinicians, professional bodies, and government. Some patients had first-hand experience of the herbal product and/or the derivatives of cannabis, so they were able to have an impact on not only the initiation of research but also its direction. They also affected the policy environment, especially as they pulled cannabis use into a more 'respectable' framework, and by keeping the issue in the minds of the press and the public they created a ground-swell of support. Through lobbying, parliamentary discussions, and submissions to key reports of the period, they kept medicinal canna-bis high on the political and scientific agenda; they also facilitated the shift from anecdotal lay knowledge to evidence-based knowl-edge with the initiation and development of clinical trials, both proof-of-principle and industrial ones. Funding was poured into the arena, and fears over the loss of the patient perspective in clinical trials led to the reinvestigation of clinical trial methodology and the development of more subtle outcome measures, which could po-tentially lead to successful outcomes in future trials.

Though lay knowledge and advocacy had an important impact on the process of remedicalization, how much actually changed from the patient perspective remained limited. The availability of a licit cannabis-based drug has often appeared to be almost within reach but never quite there. Access to CBMPs would become a significant problem and a focus of debate in later decades.

However, activism by MS associations helped change the percep-tion of cannabis so that it was no longer seen solely as a suspicious intoxicant, and many members of the public, policymakers, doc-tors, and scientists began to view cannabis as a potentially useful medicine and adjunct therapy. The voices of activists were crucial in the more open expert-committee debates of the 1990s.

6

Establishing Therapeutic Cannabis: The Role of Expert Advice, 1997–2001

The remedicalization of cannabis was shaped by the science–policy interchange. As we saw in chapter 3, private closed-committee discussions within the ACMD in the 1970s and the 1980s provided an early space for policy discussions about medicinal cannabis. This chapter further explores the importance of science–policy exchange through the public committees and the public reports on therapeutic cannabis that emerged from 1997 onwards. These reports focused specifically on the therapeutic uses of cannabis. They drew clear distinctions between cannabis's role as a medicine and its role as a recreational drug. The reports contributed significantly to the legitimatization of medical cannabis and to a shift in policymakers' attitudes towards the drug.

This chapter argues that expert advice, especially from the professional bodies in the more open committees of the late 1990s, was critical in pressuring for and facilitating clinical trials, and it moved the process of remedicalization forward. The chapter begins by looking at the initiation and the impact of the 1997 BMA report on therapeutic cannabis that cited medical needs that could be met by derivatives of cannabis. The House of Lords Science and Technology Committee report that followed a year later called for research on herbal cannabis as well as on its derivatives. These reports pressed for clinical trials, industry involvement, and a reconsideration of cannabis policy. The chapter continues by looking at how pressure mounted for permitting medical use, and at how cannabis would be rescheduled from class B to class C in 2004, following the Runciman Report of 1999 and the House of Lords follow-up report of 2001.

CANNABIS IN CONTEXT: CHANGING
ATTITUDES TO CANNABIS IN THE 1990S

Before analysing the expert advice in this later period, it is worth considering the wider environment surrounding cannabis in the late 1990s.

In the 1990s the police practice of 'cautioning' for drug possession was taking over from prosecution, and the concept of 'harm reduction' was given greater acknowledgement in policy.[1] The government deemed that public opinion was more tolerant towards cannabis. Questions in the House of Commons increased over the issue of therapeutic cannabis for sufferers of MS and cancer. MPs such as Paul Flynn, the Labour member for Newport West and a former industrial chemist, pressured for the legal medical use of cannabis, and the government received delegations on the therapeutic use of cannabis. Emphasis was placed on the outcomes of clinical trials before any modification to the MDA would be considered.[2]

The Department of Health, at the request of the ACMD, commissioned a series of unpublished literature reviews on cannabis in 1996.[3] The first review was undertaken by Professor Heather Ashton, professor of clinical psychopharmacology at the University of Newcastle-upon-Tyne, and it looked at the clinical and pharmaceutical aspects of cannabis. The second review was of the psychological and psychiatric aspects; this review was written by Dr Andrew Johns, from the Institute of Psychiatry. The third review, on the therapeutic aspects of cannabis and cannabinoids, was produced by Dr Phillip Robson, a consultant psychiatrist and senior clinical lecturer at Oxford University who went on to become medical director for GW Pharmaceuticals.[4] Paul Flynn announced his intention to ask the All-Party Parliamentary Drugs Misuse Group to back new research that would establish the risks and benefits of cannabis, with the goal of directing parliamentary opinion in favour of reform.

Nineteen ninety-seven marked a watershed for cannabis as a therapeutic. Initially, the incoming New Labour government wished to appear to take a tough stance on the drugs issue, and it appointed a US-style 'Drugs Tsar', Keith Hellawell, who was a former chief constable of West Yorkshire Police, as well as a deputy, Mike Trace, who was formerly with the Rehabilitation for Addicted Prisoners Trust. The incoming Home Secretary, Jack Straw, appeared adamantly opposed to the decriminalization of cannabis, but pressure was mounting for a re-evaluation of the situation.

Popular support for decriminalization grew, and public figures such as Paul McCartney, Richard Branson, and Anita Roddick backed a change in status. The more liberal sections of the media viewed cannabis and its legalization more positively. The *Independent on Sunday*, under the editorship of Rosie Boycott, launched the Decriminalise Cannabis campaign in September 1997 and declared that the campaign would continue 'until the law is changed and possession of marijuana for personal use is no longer an offence'.[5] The medical use of cannabis featured prominently, and the paper reported that an anonymous poll of MPs had revealed that 70 per cent favoured allowing doctors the right to prescribe cannabis for medical purposes.[6]

Senior figures within the legal system called for a reopening of the debate, including the Lord Chief Justice, Lord Bingham, who in October 1997 announced his support for open debate on the issue of legalizing cannabis. His comments were widely reported in the press. Some members of the government also began to take a softer line. The Health Secretary, Frank Dobson, reportedly said that he would consider making medical cannabis legal through a doctor's prescription. In 1998 the government launched a ten-year drug strategy that argued that resources should focus on those drugs that caused the most harm, such as heroin and cocaine.[7]

International agencies that were noted for their hostile approach to cannabis began to moderate their views about therapeutic cannabis in the 1990s. The WHO had been under pressure to review the literature on the health consequences of cannabis since the 1980s. It established an expert group on cannabis in 1993, and in December 1997 it released a report entitled 'Cannabis: Health Perspective and Research Agenda', which was aimed at policymakers and others concerned with public health.[8] The report included a section on the therapeutic use of cannabis. It also recognized that the role of derivatives had been established in the late 1970s and the early 1980s and that this had had an impact on attitudes to herbal cannabis. Although it was unenthusiastic, the WHO nevertheless considered the issues that needed to be overcome in order to study herbal cannabis: 'The therapeutic uses of THC ... have led to discussion about the therapeutic potential of cannabis itself ... To explore possible therapeutic uses ... several scientific issues need to be considered ... the standardization of cannabis preparations ... the large number of patients which would be needed to study the comparative efficacy of smoking cannabis compared with other cannabinoids and other therapeutic agents, and the possibility of using alternative delivery systems which could avoid cannabis smoking.'[9]

The WHO remained concerned, however, about the broader implications for drug control policy and also about the possible adverse effects of cannabis, particularly on mental health, but these were not considered to outweigh the potential benefits, and the report called for further research in both the laboratory and the clinic.[10] The report received more publicity than had been expected because it turned out to be rather controversial – not because of what was included but rather because of what was left out. Media reports emerged in 1998 that evidence had been suppressed after pressure was placed on the WHO by the UN International Drug Control Programme, which had been created in 1990 to improve the efficiency of the UN's drug control structure.[11] The material in question related to comparisons between cannabis and legal substances such as tobacco and alcohol. The WHO was forced to issue a rebuttal: 'There was … no attempt to hide any information and the decision not to include such a comparison in the final report was based on scientific judgment and had nothing to do with political pressure.'[12] The controversy highlighted both tensions between the agencies and the problems that cannabis posed for drug control. The comparisons between cannabis and alcohol and tobacco that had gained ground since the 1970s caused more controversy than any endorsement of therapeutic cannabis, and the issue of the relative harms of licit and illicit drugs would be revisited in domestic debates in the first decade of the twenty-first century.

In the United Kingdom concerns over the implementation of existing drug policy increased: stricter control and the increasing number of prosecutions seemed to have had a limited impact on use levels, the cost of policing was rising, and the impact on civil liberties remained a concern. But fears also remained over the relationship between cannabis and mental health, especially in light of claims of increasing THC content and uncertainty over reactions to changes in policy from the media and the public.[13] Driven by these concerns, professional bodies and expert committees began studying cannabis therapeutics between 1997 and 2004, looking at ways to advance the therapeutic use of both derivatives and herbal cannabis, and also questioning the placement of cannabis within the drug control mechanisms.

THE ROLE OF PROFESSIONAL BODIES AND
THE BRITISH MEDICAL ASSOCIATION REPORT:
'THERAPEUTIC USES OF CANNABIS', 1997

This Representative Body believes that certain additional cannabinoids should be legalized for wider medicinal use.[14]

It was against this backdrop that the BMA released its ground-breaking report on the 'Therapeutic Uses of Cannabis', adding an influential, professional, medical voice to the debate. It endorsed medical applications for the constituents of cannabis and indicated that the law surrounding them should be modified.[15]

The BMA is the UK body that represents the medical profession, and from its inception in 1832 it had commented on key issues and sought to influence public health legislation.[16] The association had an annual representatives meeting (ARM), which allowed members to debate motions, and a Board of Science and Education, which acted as the interface between the profession, the government, and the public. The board established special working parties and steering groups, and it convened outside experts for specific scientific projects. These had led to the publication of reports on a wide range of public issues, from the environmental risks of pesticides to drink-driving.[17]

A resolution was adopted at the 1994 ARM, requesting firstly that the Board of Science and Education look at the relative risks of addictive drugs and secondly that they advise on the following areas: drug misusers who wanted to break their habit; drug misusers who wished to continue; and arrangements that did, or could, exist in the future for supplying drugs to either category of drug user. A third point was also added to the resolution: to consider the benefits or otherwise of the decriminalization or legalization of some, or all, controlled drugs.[18] Sarah Mars, one of the report's authors, explained that this final request was added at the last minute: '[It] got tacked on at the end by one of the doctors at the BMA's ARM and it was agreed that they should do it.'[19]

Legalization, or decriminalization, was a controversial area for the BMA to step into. The final report explained that the BMA had refined part 3 of the resolution to refer only to controlled drugs in relation to their 'therapeutic use, by patients under medical supervision, for particular medical conditions'. Cannabis was chosen because it was of 'wide public and professional interest'.[20] In addition, the report noted that cannabis therapeutics were attracting increased interest in light of the 'increasing acceptance of herbal medicine and "natural" remedies'.[21] The report was published as a separate policy document to the larger and less-well-known BMA report titled 'The Misuse of Drugs'.[22] The fact that the report focused on therapeutics was possibly a way to assuage the issue, especially as the BMA was a cautious organization, as Sarah Mars explained: 'The Secretariat did not want to touch that issue … The BMA is a very cautious organisation. They got round it by saying they would look into the therapeutic uses of cannabis as a fudgy way of tackling the last section.'[23]

The BMA commissioned an external expert to produce a report on cannabis. Professor Roger Pertwee was asked in the first instance, due to his experience on the pharmacology of cannabis. Pertwee discussed the pharmacology of cannabis, including the newly discovered ECRS, and went on to make recommendations, including that patients with terminal illnesses should be allowed to smoke cannabis on compassionate grounds. The recommendations created controversy on several fronts: the fact that the delivery method was smoking, the use of a herbal product, and the potential press response.[24] The committee usually sent reports to two external expert referees, who forwarded their comments to the secretariat, who in turn produced the final report. Pertwee's report was sent to Professor Heather Ashton. Ashton, concerned about the possibility of the increased potency of herbal cannabis, suggested numerous changes. In light of her comments and her previous work, the committee decided to abandon Pertwee's report and instead to invite Ashton to write a more extensive one.[25]

Others who were involved in the BMA report included Professor Jack Howell, who was chair of the Board of Science and Education but who had little involvement in the report's production; Vivienne Nathanson, head of the Professional Resources and Research Group; and Dr David Morgan, head of the science department. Most of the writing was Ashton's work, but there were contributions on some points from Pertwee; Dr Anthony Moffat from the Pharmaceutical Society; Professor Patrick Wall, a pain specialist; and Sarah Mars. Clare Hodges from ACT contributed on the patient experience, and Dr William Notcutt, an anaesthetist, contributed on his experiments with nabilone for pain and MS.

The report focused on the therapeutic uses of cannabis and made eleven recommendations. In direct contrast to most of the previous reports on cannabis, it drew a distinction between therapeutic use, on which the report focused, and recreational use, which was outside its remit. The BMA committee had not previously viewed the impact of medical use on drug control as being relevant to their investigations.[26] However, this report turned the previous situation on its head. Instead of the medical use of cannabis interfering with drug control policy, drug control policy was interpreted as interfering with legitimate medical use. The report argued that the WHO should advise the CND to reschedule certain cannabinoids and that the Home Office should amend the MDA accordingly. It recognized that major amendments to international legislation were unlikely, so it instead recommended both that the government consider changing the MDA to allow the prescription of cannabinoids to patients with particular medical conditions that were not adequately treated, and that a central registry be kept of the patients to track effects over the long term.

Selected areas of research were also to be encouraged, and the pharmaceutical industry was to be drawn into the process: 'Pharmaceutical companies should undertake basic laboratory investigation and develop novel, cannabinoids analogues, and research on clinical indications for medical prescription should [be] undertaken, especially for anti-emetics, MS spinal cord injury and spastic disorders and pain, epilepsy, glaucoma, stroke and immunological effects.'[27] To reduce hindrances and facilitate research, the report indicated that the regulations should be altered: 'The regulation of cannabis and cannabinoids should be flexible to allow such compounds to be researched without [an] MDA licence issued by the Home Office.'[28]

Important questions remained over the form of cannabis and the mode of delivery. The BMA placed emphasis on cannabinoids themselves, rather than herbal products, which had unknown concentrations of cannabinoids.[29] Sarah Mars explained the cautious approach and the concern over leaf forms: 'The culture of the BMA meant they felt more comfortable with that. They were uncomfortable with leaf forms. It didn't seem scientific.'[30] The herbal product was not considered because it was the choice of recreational drug users, and nor was the use of a 'leaf' or other herbal forms considered acceptable within the context of mainstream medicine.

Critically, independent interests were drawn closer together by their mutual aim of achieving a CBM. The BMA report helped to stimulate this process by urging all stakeholders to work together to develop clinical trials: 'The Clinical Cannabinoids Group, interested patient groups, pharmaceutical companies and the Department of Health should work together to encourage properly conducted clinical trials to evaluate the further potential therapeutic uses of cannabinoids, alone or in combination, and/or in combination with other drugs.'[31] While new drugs were being developed, the report also urged the police, the courts, and the authorities to take account of medical reasons for unlawful use.

The report was released in November 1997 with an accompanying press release that was careful to distinguish between recreational and medical use but that also drew attention to some of the more emotive issues around medical cannabis use:[32] '"Therapeutic Uses of Cannabis" draws a distinction between recreational misuse and using the drug to relieve pain. The report acknowledges that thousands of people resort to taking cannabis illegally ... to ease their distressing symptoms.'[33]

The report generated considerable attention, and it had to be reprinted. It was also widely covered in the media: most coverage was positive, with headlines such as 'Doctors' Support for Cannabis'.[34] As the government had feared, some sections of the media, including the *Independent on Sunday*, linked medical arguments to policy change and reopened calls for decriminalization: 'Its appearance under the name of the BMA will give the findings added weight. It will increase pressure on the government following the launch of the *Independent on Sunday*'s campaign for the decriminalisation of cannabis and the call by the Lord Chief Justice, Sir Thomas Bingham, for a debate on the issue.'[35]

The *Independent on Sunday* used the report to add weight to decriminalization arguments, commenting: 'The publication ... of the BMA's report ... will kill off the last arguments against the decriminalisation of the drug for medical use.'[36] After the release of the report, the *Independent on Sunday* convened a conference, 'Cannabis: should it be decriminalised?', which included speakers such as Professor John Strang, the director of addiction research at the National Addiction Centre; Anita Roddick, the owner of Body Shop; Mike Goodman, a barrister and the director of Release; Professor Colin Blakemore, the chairman of the British Neuroscientific

Association; and Nigel Evans, a Conservative MP. No spokesperson from the Home Office or the BMA attended. Rosie Boycott drew attention to cannabis therapeutics in her opening speech: 'A society ... that has denied a very benign drug to MS sufferers, to recreational users, and that has made people criminals. By choosing to stick to this ... "just say no" approach we have a wildly escalating drug problem.'[37]

During the conference frequent references were made to the BMA's conclusions on therapeutic use. Austin Mitchell, a Labour MP, considered that the BMA report undermined the 1971 MDA: 'I'm open minded about the question of legalisation ... But I am concerned about the therapeutic case because in 1971 cannabis, which had been available on prescription, after that time was transferred to Schedule I of the Misuse of Drugs Act, defined as a drug which has no therapeutic value. And since then everything has been changed by this BMA report which actually says that cannabis has therapeutic value.'[38] Mitchell emphasized that a policy that led to the prosecution of patients brought the law into disrepute: 'The law's coming into disrepute, prosecutions are being abandoned, we know that the courts are imposing very lenient sentences but people still get a criminal record ... It is absolutely wrong that MS victims should be treated in that kind of fashion and driven to illegality. Something has to be done and quickly.'[39]

Prior to the conference Mitchell had taken a delegation with ACT to the Department of Health, but he found he was unable to make much progress: 'It's a chicken and egg situation in which the Home Office says it won't do anything because there is no research, but no research is done because it's illegal, and meanwhile thousands and thousands of multiple sclerosis sufferers are being forced into the backstreets into the illegal market to buy something that they know is helpful in the treatment of their condition.'[40]

The conference raised the public profile of cannabis therapeutics. The BMA report gave campaigners ammunition against government policy and it gave them the confidence to move the process of remedicalization forwards. The press picked up on splits in government over the best approach to cannabis: 'The Home Office minister George Howarth told Mr Flynn in the Commons there was no medical evidence that cannabis provided medicinal benefits. The Home Secretary Jack Straw has maintained a tough line in resisting all pressure for cannabis to be legalised, but Frank

Dobson, the Secretary of State for Health, has been more sympathetic. Mr Dobson has indicated that if medical evidence could be found, he would have no objections to cannabis being legalised for medicinal use only. Mr Flynn intends to challenge the Home Office again with the BMA findings.'[41]

The report was used both by campaigners for change and by those in favour of the status quo. For example, while the conclusion recognized the potential therapeutic value of cannabinoids, it steered clear of herbal cannabis itself, and it also recommended further research prior to access being granted.[42] The report legitimized research into cannabinoids, if not into cannabis, and provided substantial pressure for a change in legislation for medical purposes. The House of Lords report that closely followed the publication of the BMA report was able to build on the BMA's acknowledgement of potential therapeutic uses of cannabinoids, adding further pressure for action.

THE ROLE OF THE HOUSE OF LORDS SCIENCE AND TECHNOLOGY COMMITTEE: 'CANNABIS: THE SCIENTIFIC AND MEDICAL EVIDENCE', 1998

The House of Lords Science and Technology Committee report on the therapeutic use of cannabis marked a milestone in the process of remedicalization when it was published in 1998. Where the BMA had accepted therapeutic use, the Science and Technology Committee made extensive recommendations about what to do with that advice.

Select committees operate in both the House of Commons and the House of Lords, monitoring the work of government departments. The Science and Technology Committee, established in 1979, was one of the main investigative committees in the House of Lords; its inquiries were undertaken by two sub-committees. For each inquiry, members were drawn from the main committee, and additional members were chosen for their relevant expertise. At the end of an inquiry, a report, including evidence, findings, and recommendations, was presented to the main committee, and all the reports were published and debated in the House of Lords. The committee worked independently of government and was free to choose its own topics.

In February 1998 the House of Lords announced an investigation into the recreational and medical use of cannabis: this was the first time that cannabis had come under the spotlight of a select committee.[43] The report justified the decision to investigate cannabis in the context of increased interest in it following publication of the BMA report: 'In the light of this heightened interest in cannabis, and particularly the report by the BMA, we decided to examine the scientific and medical evidence to determine whether there was a case for relaxing some of the current restrictions on the medical uses of cannabis.'[44]

The interest of individual Lords was important in the selection of cannabis as a subject. Les Iversen, a retired professor of pharmacology at Oxford University and the special adviser to the cannabis committee, explained the role of disciplinary and individual interest in the choice to review cannabis: 'That group is an interesting bunch of retired scientists, doctors, lawyers, all with some interest in science and technology ... They choose a couple of topics they want to review entirely of their own initiative ... because the chairman of the sub-committee was a pharmacologist and had an interest in cannabis.'[45]

Lord Walton of Detchant, a former neurologist who had previously worked with MS patients, explained the importance to patients of the threat of prosecution: 'The Select Committee became aware that a number of well-meaning people with MS were being prosecuted.'[46] The committee approached the problem from the patient perspective rather than from concerns generated by the misuse of drugs, which had been the focus of previous expert discussions.

A sub-committee was established, with Lords members drawn from a range of disciplines but particularly from chemistry, pharmacology, and neurology; during their careers some of them had witnessed the use of cannabis by patients to treat intractable diseases. The chair, Lord Perry of Walton, was a retired professor of pharmacology from Edinburgh University who had been instrumental in the development of the Open University. Other members included Lord Porter, a Nobel Prize winning chemist; Lord Walton of Detchant; Lord Porter of Luddenham, another chemist; Lord Butterfield, a medical researcher; Lord Rea; Lord Soulsby of Swaffham Priory, an emeritus professor of animal pathology; Lord Butterworth, a lawyer and university administrator; Lord Carmichael of Kelvingrove; Lord Dixon-Smith; Lord Kirkwood, a judge; and Lord Nathan, a solicitor.

The terms of reference were wider than those of the BMA report: the committee inquired into 'the science behind the arguments over the use of cannabis and its derivatives for medical and recreational purposes'.[47] It also incorporated discussion of recreational use: 'We have also considered whether the continued prohibition of recreational use is justified on the basis of the scientific evidence of adverse effects.' However, it emphasized that it would not cover issues such as the prevalence of cannabis use, the behavioural or social aspects of drug taking, law enforcement, any relationship between drugs and crime, or the extent to which cannabis was a gateway to drug culture.[48] The report covered both cannabinoids and cannabis, and it also referred to CBMS.

Iversen drafted questions for the committee, and he was responsible for calling a wide range of witnesses.[49] Researchers such as Pertwee provided the pharmacologist's viewpoint, giving evidence of laboratory research and potential clinical applications. Clinicians, including William Notcutt, presented on clinical research, and they all provided positive feedback. Professional bodies such as the RPS and the BMA also contributed. Dr Geoffrey Guy provided the industry perspective and discussed his interest in setting up a small biotechnology company to investigate 'whole plant' cannabis. The patient perspective included the views of patients and user activists, including Clare Hodges, as well as representatives of the MS Society. Relevant government departments including the Home Office and the Department of Health provided additional witnesses. Funders such as the MRC were incorporated, as were advisory groups such as the ACMD. The committee provided an important forum to bring disparate work and perspectives under one umbrella, and its conclusions were based on a wide spectrum of stakeholders.

The report made seven recommendations to stimulate research and to change policy. The first recommendation urged that clinical trials of cannabis for the treatment of MS and chronic pain be undertaken as a matter of urgency. Support for clinical trials was not unanimous, though. Professor Griffith Edwards, who had previously sat on the ACMD committees of the 1970s, provided evidence as a witness for the ACMD along with two other psychiatrists, Malcolm Lader and Morfydd Keen. Edwards had always been wary of medical cannabis, and he queried both the value and the ethics of diverting scarce MRC funding to large-scale clinical trials, arguing against them: 'It would be reasonable to investigate the matter but I do not believe it would be reasonable to go through a controlled trial.'[50] Just as the ACMD delegation was wary of starting trials, delegates were also concerned about the misuse of drugs, should cannabis-based drugs be developed and licensed. Edwards feared the potential for the misuse of prescriptions. However, the demand for clinical trials was overwhelming from most witnesses. The Department of Health accepted the legitimacy of demands for therapeutic cannabis and appeared keen to encourage trials: 'We do see that societies such as the MS Society do have a genuine interest in the potential for therapeutic benefit ... I hope I have made it clear that the Department of Health would wish to do all it could to support and facilitate that initiative.'[51]

The MRC was brought on board to solve funding issues, and it appeared willing to speed up the process, stating: 'If there was a need for clinical trials in this area, we would be prepared to consider them out of the usual round of consideration of clinical trials.'[52] The feasibility of clinical trials was already being investigated by a new RPS working party on clinical trials protocols, and there was also involvement from GW Pharmaceuticals. With these aspects in place, the committee was keen to see trials go ahead, as Lord Walton explained: 'We did say that cannabis derivatives should continue to be controlled drugs because we did not approve [of] the so-called recreational use of cannabis ... but we were happy to approve properly designed studies of its medical use.'[53]

Two further contentious aspects were the form of cannabis to be studied and its delivery method. Conflict emerged between groups. On the one hand, the BMA, the Association of Chief Police Officers, and the Christian Institute (a charity that promoted Christianity in the United Kingdom) all supported research into the constituents of cannabis. On the other hand, those such as Dr Geoffrey Guy and Professor Wall supported research into 'whole cannabis'. The committee meeting minutes recorded the growing interest in 'whole' cannabis: 'Professor Wall argues in favour of trials of cannabis rather than pure cannabinoids. He criticises the BMA report for recommending that trials be confined to synthetic cannabinoids; he considers that it would be premature ... to assume that the only active substance in cannabis is THC.'[54]

The RPS showed support for 'whole' cannabis, and the MRC viewed a comparison as important, provided a standardized product became available. GW Pharmaceuticals made this a possibility: the company indicated its willingness and ability to produce a standardized mixture.[55] The Lords, guided by Iversen's questions, pushed the issue of research into herbal cannabis, such as when questioning witnesses. In particular, they appeared to accept the arguments of patient activists who complained about the synthetics in contrast to herbal cannabis. Subsequent clinical trials tested both synthetic THC and extracts of cannabis. GW Pharmaceuticals, the only UK company with a licence to produce CBMS, was built around the production of extracts of cannabis.

The second recommendation related to the mode of administering cannabis and the need for alternative forms: 'Research should be promoted into alternative modes of administration ... which would retain the benefits of rapid absorption offered by smoking, without the adverse effects.'[56] Modes of administration of cannabis had long been a controversial subject. The BMA had been firmly against the use of smoked cannabis. The select committee, however, did not rule out initial experiments with smoked cannabis, but it did not contemplate an eventual therapeutic based on this method and therefore pushed for the development of alternative modes of administration. Lord Walton explained: 'We could not condone smoking cannabis as we were carrying out a major campaign to ban smoking in public spaces, and there was good evidence that smoking cannabis was as potentially carcinogenic as smoking tobacco.'[57] But smoking was the method preferred by patients, and the need for a compromise stimulated research into other forms of administration, preferably one that would divide medical use from recreational use. GW Pharmaceuticals appeared to offer a solution to this problem through the development of a novel delivery system: the sublingual spray.[58]

The committee examined the impact of policy on research, and its recommendation about this aspect contributed in part to a shift in the policy environment for cannabis in subsequent years. While the committee maintained that cannabis and cannabis derivatives should remain as controlled drugs, it argued for amendments to legislation: a pragmatic approach was required to deal with patient pressure. ACT was particularly keen to see changes that would immediately impact patients, to mitigate the long, drawn-out process of research and regulation before any new drug would reach patients. Researchers also indicated that the legal situation hindered their investigations.

The committee took these concerns on board in making its recommendation, which was the most controversial in that it required the downgrading of cannabis scheduling under the MDA: a move which would have permitted the prescription of cannabis. The reported stated: 'The Government should take steps to transfer cannabis and cannabis resin from Schedule 1 of the Misuse of Drugs Regulations to Schedule 2, so as to allow doctors to prescribe an appropriate preparation of cannabis, albeit as an unlicensed medicine and on the named-patient basis and to allow doctors and pharmacists to supply the drug prescribed. This would also, incidentally, allow research without a special license from the Home Office.'[59] Amendments to the law surrounding cannabis would have allowed the prescription of cannabis-based drugs and would have had the additional advantage of creating a boundary between medical and recreational use. It was argued that such a move would support rather than weaken the drug control system: 'Legalising medical use on prescription, in the way that we recommend, would create a clear separation between medical and recreational use ... We believe it would in fact make the line against recreational use easier to hold.'[60] If the government was to contemplate a shift of cannabis from Schedule I to Schedule II, it was required by law to consult the ACMD, and therefore the fourth recommendation was to do just that. The fifth recommendation related to international policy and advised that the issue of scheduling of cannabinoids should be raised with the WHO. To counter fears over the potential diversion of prescription drugs and any link to recreational use, the final recommendation was that if doctors were permitted to prescribe cannabis on an unlicensed basis, the medical professional bodies should provide firm guidance on how to do so responsibly, and that the professional regulatory bodies should put in place safeguards to prevent the diversion to improper purposes. This would give the 'ownership' of cannabis to medical bodies.

The committee's findings were made public, and both the final report and the book of evidence were published. The government was normally expected to comment on select committee findings, so the cannabis report created a stir when it was published on 11 November 1998 and was rejected by the government on the morning of its publication. The government admitted that it had departed from the usual convention, in case its silence raised speculation that it regarded the questions around rescheduling to be open, thereby inviting hints of policy change.[61]

The government made the case that to protect patients it was not prepared to make changes prior to potential drugs passing

through the existing regulatory process, and that no interim measures would be introduced. This reaction was not unexpected;
Iversen described the response: 'The government, on [the] same
day, before the ink was dry, said they were not going to make any
changes to the law. In other words, they dismissed it out of hand.
But that was no knee jerk reaction, everyone expected that.'[62] Previous reports that had called for reclassification had been rejected.
The issue was debated in the House of Lords in December. Lord
Perry criticized the government's reaction, which appeared to
be based on concerns already addressed by the committee. Over
the issue of efficacy and safety, Lord Perry argued that cannabis
was already being used in the community and that a more pragmatic response would be to regulate such use: 'The Government
argues that prohibition protects patients ... Significant numbers
of sufferers are taking cannabis ... in defiance of the law and without medical supervision or quality control; our recommendation
would enable the health professions and the pharmaceutical industry to collaborate to provide appropriate preparations.'[63]
The select committee questioned the nature of acceptable evidence and the interpretation of that evidence. In the committee's
opinion, enough evidence already existed, even if it was largely anecdotal, and they added pressure to carry out clinical trials, which
remained the most accepted form of 'evidence'. The government's
concern that a change in legislation would reduce research was
rejected as inaccurate, and the opposite case – that research was
hindered by legislation – was put forward: 'The Government argue
that permitting prescription now would reduce the momentum of
research. On the contrary, we found evidence ... that research has
been held back by the stigma and bureaucracy associated with the
status of cannabis as an illegal drug.'[64]

Furthermore, the grounds on which the government rejected the
advice were brought into question. Firstly, if patients were the priority, on what basis should decisions be made: their safety or their
quality of life? Lord Perry argued: 'Our report shows that if cannabis is used to treat patients on the prescription of a doctor, the risk
to the patient is vanishingly small ... Many patients would regard
their safety as only their second priority after the quality of their
lives. Should not the Government share that view?'[65] Secondly, the
transparency of the rejection was questioned, with concerns being
raised over whether decisions were based on the scientific evidence

or on social grounds. Lord Perry asked: 'Is their attitude coloured by social, economic and criminological considerations to which our inquiry was not addressed? Those considerations are only pertinent to the recreational use of cannabis.'[66]

The government remained resolutely against rescheduling or prescription prior to trials, believing that 'such a move would be premature'.[67] In particular, the government argued that allowing the prescription of herbal cannabis would restrict research, and it was able to refer to the BMA's conclusions on this aspect. Nor was the government inclined to consult the ACMD, as it feared this would encourage speculation that policy change was likely when it was not: 'It would have been disingenuous to seek a view having already decided that the recommendations would not be accepted.'[68]

The government's apparently intractable position drew criticism from various quarters. Mike Pringle, chair of the council of the Royal College of General Practitioners, declared: 'I think the government is being unnecessarily cautious. The main interest here is the care of patients and the relief of patient suffering.'[69] Conflict arose over the interpretation of the phrase 'care of patients', as for some GPs it meant that, when faced with patients who had intractable disease, it was the ability to offer some treatment and relief, while for government the focus was on provision of 'safe' medicines.

The report attracted media attention. Iversen explained later that the report 'caused some interest in the conclusion that there were genuine medical uses, the dangers had been exaggerated and more research was needed'.[70] It thus reinforced the public perception that there were medical uses for cannabis and that its risks had been overstated. The media picked up on the divisions between the BMA and the House of Lords reports, especially in relation to the form of cannabis that could be used. The BBC stated: 'The BMA says it is not 100% behind a report by the House of Lords Science and Technology Committee backing the use of cannabis for medicinal purposes. The BMA, which has previously supported more clinical trials into the medical use of cannabis, says legalizing cannabis is not the answer. It believes only cannabinoids – part of the cannabis plant – should be used in medicine.'[71] But according to Iversen, the report gave the official seal of approval for medical research into cannabis. Behind the scenes, steps were being taken in regard to both therapeutic cannabis and recreational cannabis within drug policy. Lord Walton later argued that, over time, the government took note of most of the recommendations, including rescheduling: 'In general, the report was approved by government; they supported the need for further research and for reclassification of cannabis on which they consulted the ACMD.'[72]

Although the recommendation to reschedule cannabis was rejected by the government, an opening was still left for remedicalization. The report gave assurances that, if quality, safety, and efficacy could be demonstrated, cannabis would be permitted as a prescription medicine. In making the lack of clinical trial data the restraining factor, it had to facilitate clinical trials. It agreed to license trials that involved cannabis as well as cannabinoids, and the HODI was described as willing to discuss research-related licensing issues. The frail evidence base gave the government the opportunity to defer the issue, but it also meant that clinical trials of both synthetic and herbal cannabis proceeded. Those involved in the select committee claimed some responsibility for the advancement of remedicalization: 'Those involved in [the] House of Lords would like to think it was some sort of response to the fact the House of Lords said there should be more research, more proper trials ... It was a sop towards saying we were doing something towards this.'[73] Even if it was merely a sop, it still forwarded the process of remedicalization. Iversen commented: 'The report made some impact on future moves and helped stimulate the idea that there should be a proper controlled trial which the MRC took up and sponsored.'[74] Importantly, the House of Lords helped smooth the path for industry involvement that took place after 1997.[75]

The report contributed to a shift in the policy environment around cannabis generally. Certainly, some of those involved in the committee considered that it had served a useful purpose. Lord Walton commented: 'Partly as a result of our report, though I can't guarantee that, the Government downgraded cannabis.'[76] Iversen pointed out that the report came at an opportune time: 'It happened to be at a time when the Government was beginning to think about relaxing the laws on cannabis. Blunkett, the Home Secretary in 2001, suggested to the Home Office they consider the evidence for [the] downgrading of cannabis.'[77] This downgrading of cannabis, as will be discussed in more detail in the next chapter, turned out to be a short-term move, but it reflected a shift in attitudes by policymakers at the time, and it was important for facilitating medical developments.

THE UNITED KINGDOM AND
INTERNATIONAL POLICY

The government may also have been influenced by the changing attitudes of the international drug control agencies. The INCB had been hostile to cannabis since its inception under the 1961 UN Single Convention,[78] and its presidents had taken a particular interest in the mental health aspect. Hamid Ghodse, a professor of psychiatry and international drug policy at the University of London, had been a director of the International Centre for Drug Policy at St George's, University of London. He had been a member of the INCB since 1992, and had held the presidency in 1993, 1994, 1997, 1998, and 2001. He became interested in cannabis from the mental health perspective in the 1980s – an interest which he continued through his role in the international arena.[79] Despite concerns, the INCB could not ignore the developments in the medical sphere, nor the pressure for compassionate access to cannabis. Its 1998 annual report admitted that the need to investigate medical use was growing across different sectors: 'The Board is aware that there is a need to investigate ... medical use and ... there is a growing interest among the medical community, public and media.'[80]

Its changing attitudes to therapeutics may have been pragmatic, because it viewed flexibility as a means of maintaining the integrity of international drug policy. By 1998, Ghodse, then INCB president, encouraged the INCB to push for governments to carry out research into therapeutics, in order to prevent medical cannabis from being hijacked by the legalization campaigns.[81] Ghodse later explained the incentive to split the two roles of cannabis: 'To separate the political and medical aspects ... and to encourage governments to do serious, scientific research on the alleged medical usefulness of cannabis so that if its effectiveness is established, it will be a drug no different from most narcotic drugs and psychotropic substances. It can then go through the process of re-scheduling as with any other controlled medicine. If it is shown not to be effective it will not provide ammunition to those using medicine for different objectives.'[82]

However, concern remained over the relationship between cannabis medicine and recreational use: 'The Board has noted with regret how possible medical usages of cannabis have been used to justify the legalization of all cannabis use. The Board welcomes and

encourages serious scientific research on the alleged medical properties of cannabis ... but warns again misusing these research efforts
for "blanket" legalization purposes.'[83]

Evolving perceptions of cannabis appeared to have the power to
disrupt the entire drug classification framework. In contrast to comparisons that were emerging of cannabis with socially acceptable,
licit drugs such as alcohol and tobacco, the INCB found it important to maintain cannabis's close ties to controlled, narcotic drugs:
'Should the medical usefulness of cannabis be established it will be
a drug no different to most narcotic drugs and psychotropic substances. This means that cannabis used for medical purpose would
be subject to licensing and other control measures foreseen under
the international drug control treaties.'[84]

Ghodse's view was that the INCB stance gave the green light for
research and stimulated studies in the United Kingdom, such as
the MRC clinical trials.[85] Researchers in the United Kingdom, on the
other hand, denied that the INCB standpoint – or indeed that of any
of the international agencies – had much impact.[86] Was it rather
that the INCB wanted to catch up with events that had moved beyond its ability to control?

The UK government's tone, if not its policy, was changing. Clinical trials and industry involvement moved forward in the United
Kingdom after the House of Lords report, and the following
years saw the establishment of clinical trials and attempts to license cannabis-based drugs; in the process, these developments
contributed to wider drug policy debates. But while the process
of remedicalization was moving forward, potential changes to the
drug classification system proved to be more problematic.

RESCHEDULING CANNABIS: 'DRUGS AND
THE LAW: REPORT OF THE INDEPENDENT INQUIRY
INTO THE MISUSE OF DRUGS ACT 1971'

The issue of medical cannabis became more politicized, integrating
with calls for rescheduling in expert reports. One of the landmark
reports that focused on the rescheduling debate was 'Drugs and the
Law: Report of the Independent Inquiry into the Misuse of Drugs
Act 1971', otherwise known as the Runciman Report, released in
1999.[87] This aimed to tackle issues that the previous House of Lords
report had not covered.

In August 1997 the Police Foundation, with the assistance of the Prince's Trust, established a committee chaired by Viscountess Runciman, a long-standing member of the ACMD, the chair of the council's Criminal Justice Working Group, and the chair of the Mental Health Act Commission. Members included representatives from drug service organizations, such as Alison Chesney, chief executive of the Cranston Drug Services; from the legal profession, including Rudi Forston, a barrister-at-law, Middle Temple, and a founding member of Release; from the police service, including John Hamilton, the chief constable of Fife Constabulary; and from academe, including Professor David Nutt, head of the Mental Health and Psychopharmacology Unit at the University of Bristol. Other committee members included Simon Jenkins, the former editor of *The Times*; Ian Wardle, the chief executive of Lifeline Project Limited; and Annette Zera, the principal of Tower Hamlets College, London.

The committee reviewed the 1971 MDA. It argued that the classification system needed to be more closely related to the scientific evidence of relative harm. Cannabis was the focus of one chapter, in which it was considered in relation to the harms of other illicit drugs, and the committee concluded that cannabis was less harmful than those other drugs and that the current law was therefore problematic: 'If our drugs legislation is to be credible, effective and able to support a realistic programme of prevention and education, it has to strike the right balance between cannabis and other drugs.'[88]

The committee concluded that there was little evidence that the law was effective as a deterrent. Like the ACMD before it, it urged reclassification of cannabis from class B to class C and from Schedule I to Schedule II of the regulations of the MDA – a move that would allow supply and possession for medical purposes. Within the discussion of cannabis, therapeutic use played an important part in relation to its impact on the MDA:

> We conclude that there is evidence that there are
> therapeutic benefits from the use of cannabis by people
> with certain serious illnesses and that these benefits
> outweigh any potential harm to themselves. We therefore
> agree with the House of Lords Select Committee that
> cannabis and cannabis resin, together with tincture and

extracts not covered by the 1971 Convention, should be
transferred from Schedule I to Schedule II to the 1985
regulations. That would automatically ensure that doctors
who prescribed such substances were not criminally liable.
The same would apply to their patients in possession and
doctors or pharmacists who supplied cannabis.[89]

The committee had little to add to the conclusions of the BMA
and the House of Lords report other than to endorse and further
their recommendations: 'We appreciate the doubts of the BMA over
how to control and assess dosages of raw cannabis. But these seem
to us insufficient reasons for preventing prescription where doctors,
at their own risk on a named-patient basis, believe that their patients
will benefit.'[90]

In light of the medical conditions for which medical cannabis was
being investigated, attitudes to the form and the delivery methods
of cannabis were also undergoing change: 'While understanding
the reservations expressed by the British Medical Association and
the House of Lords Select Committee about administration by
smoking, this seems to us a very minor matter given the seriousness
of the conditions for which prescription of cannabis seems likely to
be beneficial.'[91]

The report called for immediate changes prior to the results of
clinical trials. It rejected one government fear – that of the misuse
of prescriptions – and noted that the ability to prescribe heroin for
pain relief had not caused a problem: 'We do not share the Government's anxiety about the capacity of GPs to withstand pressure
for the prescription of cannabis. There is no evidence that this has
been a problem where the prescription of heroin for pain control
is concerned.'[92]

The Runciman Committee built on the House of Lords demands
for compassionate access to medical cannabis and called for a legal defence based on medical grounds: 'As the Government has
rejected the House of Lords recommendations and it will be some
years before a standard licensed cannabis product is available, we
recommend that there should be a new defence of duress of circumstances on medical grounds for those accused of possessing,
cultivating or supplying cannabis ... This approach would comply
with our international obligations under the United Nations conventions and enable spurious defences to be rejected.'[93]

The committee reported their conclusions in March 2000, but the Home Secretary, Jack Straw, rejected reclassification. He did promise, however, that the remaining recommendations would receive serious consideration. Meanwhile, the report received considerable media attention and was generally well received. *The Independent* newspaper, unsurprisingly given its previous line on cannabis, reported the dismissive government response, as did the BBC.[94] The House of Commons Home Affairs Select Committee pressured for a full response from the Home Secretary, but when the government responded in full in February 2001 it rejected most of the key recommendations. Viscountess Runciman expressed her confidence in the enduring quality of the report: 'Our recommendations on cannabis were by far the most far-reaching and they were meant to be, because we think that that is where the law is, in a sense, most defective ... This is a good report, [it] has staying power and ... its time will come.'[95] She appeared confident that the recommendations would stand the test of time and that policy change would be implemented at an opportune moment. When the report was discussed by the Home Affairs Select Committee in June 2000, it came in for criticism over its independence and its 'soft' view on drugs.[96] Runciman was scathing about the government's response, claiming that the law caused more harm than it stopped: 'It also leaves us with a law that in relation to cannabis produces more harm than it prevents.'[97]

Pressure continued to build for a rethink of drug policy and drug regulation. Therapeutic aspects of cannabis were again in the headlines, due to the release of the second House of Lords inquiry into therapeutic cannabis in March 2001, a follow-up inquiry to their 1998 report.[98] This inquiry covered research that had taken place since the initial report, but it also dealt with the legal situation and the growing concerns over the prosecution of patients who were using cannabis medically. The terms of reference were to 'examine the current state of research into the therapeutic uses of cannabis, the roles of the Home Office and the Medicines Control Agency in the licensing of CBMs, and more recent issues relating to the prosecution of therapeutic cannabis users'.[99]

The 2001 report reiterated the points made in the 1998 report, but with clinical trials underway for the first time, the role of regulatory and licensing bodies came under scrutiny. Once again the reconsideration of regulatory requirements was urged. At that point there was more receptiveness to the concept. The report referred to an apparent change in attitude by the government to the prescription of CBMs: 'We are pleased to note that the Government now displays a more encouraging attitude towards the licensing of therapeutic preparations of cannabis ... In effect, the Minister assured us that once a safe, effective, CBM had been licensed by the Medicines Control Agency, the Government would actively cooperate in permitting it to be prescribed.'[100]

The long timescale for the licensing of CBMs was deemed to relate to the fear that medical use might stimulate greater recreational use rather than to objections to medical cannabis itself: 'Up until now we have sensed that the authorities have been dragging their feet, at least partly because they may have feared that permitting therapeutic preparations of cannabis to be prescribed would be interpreted by the public as a move towards allowing recreational use.'[101]

But by 2001 the government had come to view the remedicalization of cannabis as a means to provide a clear distinction between medical use and non-medical use. The development of clear medical and non-medical structures for cannabis would weaken calls for decriminalization and would make it easier for the government to clamp down on recreational use if required: 'There is now a much sharper awareness of the distinction between medicinal use of cannabis and recreational use of cannabis in the public debate ... We are pleased, too, that the Minister now shares our view that, were the law relaxed on the therapeutic use of cannabis, the Government's hand in suppressing illegal, recreational use would be strengthened.'[102]

But the House of Lords had concerns over this stage of the process of remedicalization. The progress in clinical trials was slow, and it appeared that the need for licences, and the continued stigma around cannabis, still inhibited research. In the meantime, it was considered undesirable to prosecute therapeutic cannabis users. In addition, there were fears that the MCA had failed to take a balanced, objective view of cannabis-based drugs and that it needed to reconsider its position. The House of Lords Report explained:

> We are concerned that the MCA's approach to the licensing
> of cannabis-based medicines, and their insistence on the
> provision of new toxicological data which could delay
> the approval of such medicines, place the requirements

of safety and the needs of patients in an unacceptable balance. Patients with severe conditions … are being denied the right to make informed choices about their medication. There is always some risk in taking any medication; patients and their doctors should certainly be informed about the toxicological concerns that the MCA have raised, but these concerns should not prevent them from having access to what promises to be the only effective medication available to them. Overall, we consider that the MCA's attitude means that cannabis-based medicines are not being dealt with in the same impartial manner as other medicines.

The positive response of the Lords to cannabis did not go unnoticed, capturing the attention of the press, which produced headlines such as 'Lords Back Cannabis Use'.[103]

The general election in June 2001 saw the re-election of the Labour government. The new government seemed more inclined to reconsider cannabis, and in July 2001 the incoming Home Secretary, David Blunkett, was reported as wanting to reopen the drug debate. Pressure mounted when, in July 2001, the Home Affairs Select Committee announced its intention to hold an inquiry entitled 'The Government's Drugs Policy: Is It Working?' Later that year came an indication that policy change might be underway. At a Home Affairs Select Committee meeting, Blunkett announced that he favoured the reclassification of cannabis and asked the ACMD to review the classification in the light of the scientific evidence. At the meeting he made it clear that, subject to the satisfactory outcome of the clinical trials, he would approve a change to the Misuse of Drugs legislation to enable the prescription of a CBM: 'Should this programme be proved to be successful, I will recommend to the Medicines Control Agency that they should go ahead with authorising the medical use of this for medical purposes. In the event of the successful completion of clinical trials and a positive evaluation by the MCA, we recommend that the law is changed to permit the use of cannabis-based medicines.'[104]

The Home Affairs Select Committee signalled its agreement that the dangers of cannabis relative to other drugs had been overstated and that the greater public health danger might lie in the loss of credibility of the entire drug control system: 'Whether or not cannabis is a gateway drug, we do not believe there is anything to be gained by exaggerating its harmfulness. On the contrary, exaggeration undermines the credibility of messages that we wish to send regarding more harmful drugs. We support, therefore, the Home Secretary's proposal to reclassify cannabis from class B to class C.'[105]

While these moves to reclassify cannabis were taking place, therapeutic issues were also brought back to the table, and the government response to each of the House of Lords reports' recommendations was released in December 2001. The government reiterated its encouragement of clinical trials: 'The Government has consistently made it clear that it welcomes clinical trials into the therapeutic use of cannabis ... This remains the position.'[106] The government appeared to take a relaxed attitude to the fact that the criminal justice system was taking a sympathetic view of medical users of cannabis, stating: 'While the law can make no distinction on the criminality of the possession of cannabis for recreational or therapeutic reasons, while the efficacy and safety of the latter remain unproved, the Government believes that the criminal justice system does allow for a sympathetic approach to the genuine therapeutic user.'[107] They went on to defend the MCA and the regulatory process:

> The Government accepts that it should be impartial in
> its approach to licensing cannabis-based medicines ...
> Development of cannabis-based medicines poses a number
> of very difficult scientific and regulatory problems. The
> MCA is treating these products in the same way as any other
> drug, taking account of all the information available on
> the balance of risks and benefits including relevant human
> exposure, in making their decisions. Whilst acting within
> the appropriate constraints of regulations that protect
> clinical trials subjects, the MCA is working closely with
> those developing these products to identify solutions to
> the specific problems. In doing so the MCA has contributed
> significantly to the progress of the development of these
> medicines.[108]

The ACMD presented its report to the Home Secretary in March 2002, recommending that all cannabis products be reclassified as class C and that they be moved from Schedule I to Schedule II of the MDA 1985 regulations, on the grounds that cannabis was less harmful than other substances within class B. The report made reference to a possible link between the chronic use of cannabis and mental illness, but it stated that 'no clear causal link has been demonstrated'. The impact on therapeutic cannabis was that it was now split from the drugs debate, indicating that it could be treated as a separate issue: 'The Council is aware, however, that clinical trials of cannabis derivatives are in progress. If, at some future date, one or more cannabis preparations become available as medicinal substances then the Council would advise about which Schedule, under the Misuse of Drugs Regulations 2001, they should be categorized. This matter, however, is entirely separate from the classification of cannabis under the MDA 1971.'[109] This time the government would follow the ACMD's advice. These debates would ultimately lead to the downgrading of cannabis in 2004 but, for the time being, all eyes switched to the outcome of the clinical trials, which are discussed in detail in the following chapter.

CONCLUSION

A major alteration in attitudes took place towards cannabis in the period between 1997 and 2001. Research and anecdotal reports filtered through to expert committees and professional organizations, which released positive reports, and the concept of cannabis as a medicine rapidly replaced the concept of cannabis as a menace. These professional bodies and expert committees conferred a new level of legitimacy on cannabis's therapeutic potential during this period, encouraged a shift in attitude, and increased demands for rescheduling.

As pressure mounted, national and international agencies eased restraints on medical research, in order to enable the creation of a divide between medical and recreational use. Funding and incentives again flowed into the field. Concerns shifted to focusing on the form of cannabis that would be utilized and its delivery methods. But the debates also opened up questions about the roles and functions of the international control agencies and drug control policies. Clinical trials were seen as the way forward, and they facilitated a reduction in uncertainty over cannabis's therapeutic potential and provided a clear split between licit medical use and illicit recreational use. The early 2000s would see the remedicalization of cannabis hinge on the outcomes of clinical trials.

From Anecdotal to Evidence-Based Medicine: The Role of Clinical Trials, 1995–2005

Randomized controlled trials (RCTs) are the benchmark in biomedicine, and cannabis had to be a success in clinical trials if it was to become a licensed medicine again.

Historians and social scientists have given various reasons for the growth of the RCT: the development of statistics; the advent of experimental epidemiology; the professional and organizational interests of the MRC; the relative importance of key individuals, including Bradford Hill; and, lastly, fears over medical technology in the 1970s encouraging the funding of RCTs.[1] Rosser Mathews has placed the birth of modern clinical trials in the context of the search for quantification. He has revealed how the merging of statistics and medicine was an attempt to move medical decision-making away from an art and towards a science.[2]

Clinical trial methodology became increasingly sophisticated, from the addition of randomization, to 'double blinding', and to crossover trials. British medical researchers such as Archie Cochrane encouraged the more effective use of medical resources through techniques such as RCTs.[3] Historians have shown how clinical trials impacted health policy, as well as the provision of therapeutics. Meldrum has demonstrated how RCTs became a tool of policymaking in the United States, where clinical trials became the route for passing medicine through the newly established FDA in the post-thalidomide era.[4]

All that said, clinical trials have not been without their critics. Ethical considerations have always been important, ranging from the ethics of withholding potential treatment to concerns over the safety of participants when pushing at medical frontiers. Other researchers have voiced concerns about outcome measures, especially in studies of pain, while postmodernists have contended that trials cannot be truly objective as they are linked with their social context. For instance, Troth's PhD thesis on the history of clinical trials shows how concerns have been raised over ethics, e.g. the problems of outcome measures, particularly in studies of pain. Troth also notes the postmodernist argument that trials cannot be truly objective, as they are influenced by their social context, citing investigations into analgesics in particular.[5]

Clinical trials of THC tablets in the United States in the 1970s moved cannabis away from anecdotal medicine and towards evidence-based medicine. In the 1980s these trials led to the licensing of Marinol (dronabinol) and Cesamet (nabilone) as anti-emetics and/or appetite stimulants. These drugs had limited uptake and were largely superseded by other medicines for these uses, but the process set a precedent. Until 2000 reports on cannabis's medical use remained largely anecdotal or dependent on single-case reports, or at best small-scale clinical trials. Herbal cannabis was not considered in these trials, all of which investigated THC.

This chapter charts the growing interest in cannabis in UK clinical trials from different stakeholders, and the convergence of interest in the 1990s that saw a collective desire to see the production of additional cannabis-based drugs. Two avenues opened up: one was an academic route, with 'proof-of-principle' trials; and the other was through GW Pharmaceuticals, who wanted to license cannabis extracts.[6]

These developments led to large-scale, double-blind RCTs. These had mixed outcomes, demonstrating the difficulties of clinical cannabis research, which was compounded by symptoms that were complicated to measure, such as pain. General issues that were specific to clinical trials, such as recruitment and retention, all proved problematic. Trials were an important step in the process of remedicalization, reducing some aspects of uncertainty and demonstrating some efficacy and safety, but they did not lead to easy access for patients.

THE IMPORTANCE OF CLINICAL
TRIAL METHODOLOGY

Clinical trials are broken down into four phases. Phase I establishes how a medicine works and its dosage, with the medicine administered to healthy volunteers. Phase II tests safety and efficacy on small groups of patients with the relevant illness. Phase III tests safety and efficacy in large groups of patients. Phase IV is a post-licensing phase. If the drug successfully passes through the first three phases, it would normally be approved by a national regulatory authority.

In the United Kingdom this regulatory authority is the MHRA (known as the MCA until 2003). If a medicine is shown to be safe and effective, the MHRA licenses the drug and provides marketing authorization (previously known as a product licence). In making regulatory and licensing decisions, advice is sought from an advisory committee called the Commission on Human Medicines (the Medicines Commission and the Committee on Safety of Medicines prior to 2005).

In the 1980s the harmonization of clinical trial protocols across the EU was shown to be feasible. Moreover, coordination between Europe, Japan, and the United States led to a joint regulatory–industry initiative on international harmonization known as the International Council on Harmonisation of Technical Requirements for Registration of Pharmaceuticals for Human Use.

Above and beyond the difficulties of researching a controlled substance, the RCT presented a specific set of issues for cannabis. While discussing psychopharmacology, Healy has argued that not all drugs are easily amenable to that form of evidence-based medicine: 'The match between drug therapies and RCTs is based on the idea that a drug embodied one active principle which had been isolated and could be delivered systematically.'[7] He has illustrated how not all drugs could be considered within the framework of 'magic bullets', and they are instead complex cocktails of compounds containing a number of therapeutic principles.[8] These issues were pertinent to the progress of cannabis through the licensing system. As a highly complex plant substance, it was difficult for researchers to ascertain the form of cannabis that they should research and develop. Up to the 1990s the only area that had been seriously investigated was THC, which led to the licensing of nabilone and dronabinol, but these drugs failed to fulfil expectations, partly because they were heavily restricted and partly because patients appeared to prefer

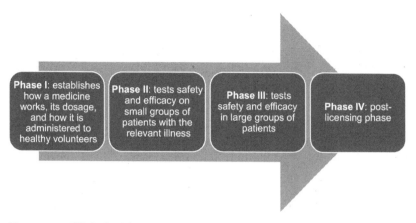

Figure 7.1 Clinical trials stages.

herbal cannabis. In this context the door opened to research not only on something more akin to cannabis itself, but also for additional applications of cannabis.

THE INITIATION OF CLINICAL TRIALS ON CANNABIS IN THE UNITED KINGDOM, 1995–2000

Research had begun to support anecdotal evidence of cannabis's therapeutic role, especially with the discovery of the ECRS. Interest shifted from the laboratory to the clinic, giving a new legitimacy to cannabis. There was already anecdotal evidence of cannabis's benefits in the treatment of MS and pain, and in the mid-1990s clinical interest was focused on this area. MS had few treatments, and no new drug for pain had been introduced in twenty years. Only six trials for MS, with a total of forty-one patients, had been previously carried out: this was insufficient for considering the licensing of CBMs.

The interest of specific individual clinicians was a key factor in the research focus of trials. The clinicians who led the trials had had an early interest in MS and/or pain and had witnessed how patients smoked herbal cannabis to alleviate their symptoms. Professor John Zajicek, who led an MRC-funded trial on MS, was a neurologist with a PhD on the cell biology of MS. In 1995, after moving to Plymouth, he became involved in the clinical aspects of MS.

Another clinician who began trials on MS and pain was Dr William Notcutt. Notcutt had qualified in Birmingham in 1970, and he had come across cannabis being used as a bush tea for alcoholism and glaucoma while working at the University of the West Indies in Kingston, Jamaica. In 1982 he moved to the James Paget Hospital at Great Yarmouth as a consultant anaesthetist, where he focused on chronic pain. He set up a palliative care service in 1985 and introduced patient-controlled analgesia for patients with post-operative pain. In looking at the history of pain treatment, he had come across references to cannabis and had observed patients self-medicating with the drug. In 1994 he accompanied patients and Professor Patrick Wall, an eminent pain specialist, to parliament to campaign for patient access to medicinal cannabis. Notcutt began testing nabilone on patients suffering from pain and MS when the drug became available on a named-patient basis.[9]

Dr Anita Holdcroft was another clinician who had come across the use of cannabis by patients, and she had investigated its usefulness prior to the development of the major clinical trials. Her focus was on acute pain rather than MS. She was an anaesthetist who had worked in West Africa in the 1980s; on her return to the United Kingdom in the early 1990s she retrained in pain medicine and set up a pain clinic at the Hammersmith Hospital. It was an era when the science of pain medicine was emerging, and her interest in cannabinoids was triggered when she found herself dealing with 'very limited management strategies' for problems that were inadequately described or that had inadequate treatments.[10] Although she had read of advances in pain management, she found that they were not put into practice in the clinical environment, so she took it upon herself to develop small-scale trials.

Holdcroft had one patient who suffered from familial Mediterranean fever (an inflammatory condition of the gut) who used cannabis to reduce his symptoms. On discussion with the patient it was decided that Holdcroft would develop a clinical trial.[11] The trial took a year to initiate. The patient had been prescribed oral morphine, but they self-treated with herbal cannabis. Holdcroft struggled to obtain cannabis for the trial. Marinol was difficult to import, and Holdcroft was aware that the patient preferred herbal cannabis anyway. Fred Evans, professor of pharmacognosy at the School of Pharmacy, worked on inflammation and was able to provide small amounts of cannabis in the form of a capsule. The MS Society, wary of the drug's illegal status, refused to fund the study. By contrast, the Home Office appeared keen on the trial and wanted it to be scaled up; this proved to be infeasible, as finding other suitable patients was problematic.

The trial revealed issues that also proved to be a problem with later clinical trials. For example, Holdcroft's patient could obtain cannabis off the street, and he knew that it helped with his pain. On the placebo he therefore became irritable, and he had to be persuaded to remain in the trial. This issue of retention would re-occur with a vengeance in later trials. But despite these problems the results of the trial were positive. The drug showed anti-inflam-matory properties, and Holdcroft was able to demonstrate that cannabis use reduced the amount of morphine that was required to control pain.[12]

This was only a very small-scale trial, however ($n = 1$): the study of one patient was not proof on its own. That said, some research-ers have argued that $n = 1$ trials, such as those used in psychological research, might be a suitable alternative method to the favoured large-scale trials.[13] Nevertheless, the United Kingdom gained expe-rience in the application of cannabis for MS and pain. Moffat noted that trials were largely too small: 'The clinical trials that had been carried out were either too small (20–30 patients) or had no real objective end points.' Pressure for large-scale trials therefore grew.[14] The nebulous qualities of these health problems, together with the complex therapeutic under investigation, had both benefits and complications for clinical trials and for the licensing of any poten-tial cannabis-based drugs.

Clinicians' individual research interests were pulled together by professional bodies in the mid-1990s. By that stage the professional organizations were prepared to become involved in cannabis re-search, and both their influence and their expertise facilitated the initiation of large-scale clinical trials. In 1995 the council of the RPS (the regulatory and professional body for pharmacists in England, Scotland, and Wales) took an active role in stimulating cannabis research. The society issued a statement noting that more clinical research was needed to investigate the potential therapeutic uses of cannabinoids in specific medical conditions. It suggested that, due to the time lag before research results, there was a case for allow-ing doctors to prescribe cannabinoids for serious named disorders.

To this end, the Pharmaceutical Sciences Group from the RPS, in conjunction with the MS Society and with the support of the BMA, arranged a public meeting entitled 'The Therapeutic Applications

of Cannabinoids'. The meeting was attended by more than 130 people and was held at the School of Pharmacy in March 1997. The
goal of the meeting was to survey the evidence for the medical use
of cannabinoids; to review the history, chemistry, and pharmacology
of cannabinoids; and to clarify the legal position on using cannabinoids therapeutically.[15] The meeting highlighted the need and
pressure for research into medical cannabis. Dr Anita Holdcroft recalled: 'Different vocal groups were there. They strongly advocated
the medicinal use of cannabis. We could see that some patients were
getting value out of it. There were concerns ... they had no idea of
the doses. They were probably taking too much.'[16]

Since medical use of herbal cannabis already existed in the patient
community, one justification for trials was to ascertain an efficacious
and safe dosage, and the March 1997 meeting was a catalyst for the
development of clinical trials. Anthony Moffat, who was from the
RPS and who was a professor at the School of Pharmacy, described
how discussions at the end of the meeting stimulated his interest in
moving the process forward: 'Anita Holdcroft and I were there together with the dean of the School of Pharmacy, and she said: "Why
doesn't somebody do some clinical trials?" ... I thought: "Well, she's
absolutely right."'[17] But the question was whether trials were feasible in the political climate. Moffat, from the School of Pharmacy,
and Vivienne Nathanson, from the BMA, met with Kenneth Cal-
man, Chief Medical Officer for England, who agreed that it was a
good time to do trials.[18] Alan Macfarlane, the Chief Inspector of the
Home Office Drugs Branch, indicated that a study would be viewed
favourably, but he stressed the necessity for good-quality proposals.

In order to develop such proposals, the Clinical Cannabinoid
Working Group, under the auspices of the RPS, put informal networks of interested researchers – such as the Clinical Cannabinoid
Group convened by Dr Pertwee – on a more formal footing. The
group was chaired by Professor Sir William Asscher, the former
chairman of the Committee on Safety of Medicines, and it included
representation from the NHS research and development directorate,
the MRC, the MS Society, as well as individual researchers including
Professor Pertwee, Dr Zajicek, Dr Anita Holdcroft, and Dr William
Notcutt. Moffat explained the nature of the RPS's involvement: 'The
Society has a long-standing involvement with research into the medicinal benefits of cannabis and the publication of this work shows
that cannabis has some therapeutic effect in the treatment of MS.

The Society's policy on cannabinoids (the active constituents of cannabis) was to see clinical trials undertaken to show the therapeutic benefits.'[19] The working group met in July and August 1998 with a clear remit: to prove the value of cannabis, not to bring a drug to market. As Sir William Asscher explained: 'We were quite insistent we would have no involvement in the development of drugs, merely the proof of principle.'[20]

The objectives of the working group were to produce guidelines that future trials could follow, with the aim of speeding up and facilitating the process of approving and funding trials, trial development, and the publication of results. The group met a number of times over the course of eighteen months to hammer out potential trial designs.[21] Clinical trial designs and objectives were written into a document called a clinical trial protocol. The protocol acted as the 'operating manual' and ensured that researchers in different locations performed a given trial in a similar way on patients with similar characteristics – this was essential in multi-centre trials.

Those eighteen months proved to be a significant period in the process of remedicalizing cannabis, because, as chapter 6 demonstrated, events were taking place that were changing the environment around cannabis and that smoothed the path for clinical trials. Cannabis's illegal status provided political pressure and a flow of funding for research into cannabis that many potential legal medicines did not attract. Zajicek commented on the auspicious timing of the trials: 'It was luck really. A time when there were a number of factors that all conspired together. There was a big push to make cannabis legal. The government wanted to test new treatments. New Labour didn't want to legalize. They wanted it to be tested. They were keen on getting results through scientific evidence.'[22]

As discussed in chapter 5, patient experience and patient advocacy played an important role in the stimulation of trials. The patient perspective was particularly important when it came to pain management. Holdcroft elaborated on the significance of pain and MS in terms of the flexible attitudes in the United Kingdom towards cannabis: 'In pain you listen to what a patient tells you … it's very much a subjective assessment. So, it seemed reasonable to follow up on their experience. It was also what MS people were saying. [It] only really happened in this country … I think it was because there was some latitude in the use of cannabis.'[23] She also recalled: 'There was quite a lot of activity through the MS Society. They were starting really to lobby.'[24] User activism and pressure, combined with the government's interpretation of the international conventions, meant that it was possible for clinical trials to go ahead.

FUNDING AND THE ROLE OF THE MEDICAL RESEARCH COUNCIL

The government was keen to support research that could provide a licit CBM and that could eliminate the medical argument for the legalization of cannabis, but to do this it was necessary to have a better evidence base. Zajicek has argued that the illicit nature of cannabis and the subsequent pressure from the government helped direct funds into cannabis: 'We are lucky in that it's got a high profile in that it's a drug of abuse. If it wasn't, I don't know if we would have funding now. I have a lot of colleagues that want to do clinical trials and can't. You need to have reasons to do one ... having politicians on your back is useful. It's good for us to some extent.'[25]

Undertaking a clinical trial is an expensive and complicated process. The support that was provided by the MRC was important both financially and to ease the burden of multi-centre trials. As Zajicek commented: 'We didn't have funding. So we approached the MRC. They were helpful in trying to make sure grant applications were successful ... and in facilitating the co-ordination of the study.'[26]

The MRC was reorganized during this period, and the cannabis trials benefited from the organization's new structure. The MRC Clinical Trials Unit (CTU) was formed in October 1998 to continue research programmes in HIV and cancer as well as continuing activities in statistical methodology, meta-analysis, and quality of life research. The CTU, directed by Professor Janet Darbyshire, aimed to initiate trials in new areas in which there were important questions to answer but where there was either insufficient infrastructure or few clinical trials. An MRC Trial Development Group advised applicants on cannabis trial designs to ensure that applications were highly competitive in obtaining funding.

The MRC also participated in the RPS's working party on therapeutic uses of cannabis. This group reported to the House of Lords committee that there was a shortage of high-quality research proposals on cannabis, and it indicated that it would be supportive of funding clinical trials and would consider grant applications out of turn in order to speed up the process. The RPS stated: 'It is particularly important that the potential for new medicinal drugs ... is not stifled by considering all cannabis-like compounds as medically unacceptable because of the abuse potential of the natural product ... The MRC would be supportive of funding well-conceived clinical trials ... It is important to evaluate in a rigorous manner whether cannabis or cannabinoids do indeed offer any relief of symptoms in neurological disease.'[27] Holdcroft cited the significant role of the House of Lords in encouraging the MRC to fund trials: 'The House of Lords put pressure on the MRC to do this study because they recommended trials. Normally trials are done by a pharmaceutical manufacturer rather than government and the MRC doesn't normally fund them unless for specific purposes.'[28] The result was that Zajicek's trial on cannabinoids in multiple sclerosis (CAMS) received an initial £1.5 million from the MRC, and that Holdcroft's trial on cannabis for acute post-operative pain (CANPOP) received £500,000 from the MRC. Shortfalls were sought from specific-disease charities such as the MS Society.

THE DEVELOPMENT OF CLINICAL TRIALS:
CANNABIS FORM, SUPPLY, AND ADMINISTRATION

A major question for the trials was which form of cannabis to study. Both industry and proof-of-principle trials incorporated the study of cannabis extracts as well as of synthetic THC. GW Pharmaceuticals grew its own cannabis, and it solved the problem of standardization and supply when it developed an oral-mucosal spray based on extracts of herbal cannabis. For the proof-of-principle trials, much debate took place over the forms of cannabis to trial. As Zajicek explained: 'We had to work out which drugs we were going to use. We knew that THC was likely to be the most active ingredient. THC was already being used because in [the] United States it had a licence in the form of Marinol for nausea related to cancer chemotherapy ... If THC worked, we would be able to get it out quickly because it was already being manufactured and used. We wanted to put THC in there. But if it didn't work and there was something else in cannabis then we would be criticized so we had to include an arm with a cannabis extract.'[29] For reasons of practicality the trials were focused mainly on THC: Marinol was an obvious choice, and Unimed supplied it free of charge.

By using extracts of cannabis, these trials therefore marked a new avenue for clinical trials. This was not without controversy, as the use of an extract posed concerns. Some feared the potential diversion of use, and others, such as Professors Ashton and Nathanson from the BMA, were against the use of material other than a synthetic single chemical entity on the grounds that a botanical extract was a complex substance with unknown effects. Zajicek highlighted some of the difficulties: 'It's very difficult to identify every last component. THC is manufactured so we know what is in there. In an extract from a plant there are tens of different cannabinoids and all other things such as flavinoids.'[30]

Nevertheless, pressure was mounting for evidence-based research in something that was more akin to the herbal cannabis with which patients self-medicated. GW Pharmaceuticals had decided to go down the extract route, and Professor Asscher's working group was keen to see this area investigated, believing that it was possible 'to overcome problems of standardization, and reap benefits of the whole plant'.[31] Professor Wall was also in favour of the investigation of an extract, and he criticized the BMA's position of testing only synthetic cannabinoids. Support for an extract came from a diverse array of parties: the RPS; individual researchers, including Professor Roger Pertwee; and patient groups, such as ACT, whose members were already using herbal cannabis, and the MS Society, which wanted to test all options. Holdcroft explained why those interested in pain wanted to pursue an extract: 'We were starting to know what compounds were in the plant. There was a big lobby to use the plant rather than THC. For pain it was obvious you needed to use more than one drug … as long as we knew what was in it.'[32]

Technological progress facilitated trials of cannabis extracts. The advent of mass spectrometry techniques in the 1980s weakened the original argument that it was not possible to define what was in a plant. Indeed, a mixture of substances was seen as potentially advantageous, especially for pain and MS. On this basis, the protocols incorporated one arm that explored the effects of 'whole' cannabis.

The provision of an extract was more complicated than the provision of THC. The School of Pharmacy had produced cannabis under the guidance of Fred Evans, who had grown cannabis for the Home Office. However, it was not geared up to provide the quantity needed for multi-centre clinical trials – such large quantities were usually provided by industry. Furthermore, standardization remained an issue. Initially, it was hoped that GW Pharmaceuticals might provide the product for the extract arm of the protocols, but financial and practical constraints intervened. Zajicek met Guy in the 1990s and discussed a supply of material, but GW was in its formative stages at that time, and it did not have a product to commit to the trials. In addition, Guy would have required payment,[33] but the low or zero cost of research material was important in the 1970s.

The presentation of the protocols at an RPS meeting in 1999 provided an opportunity to introduce the project to interested companies. The German charity the European Centre for Immunological and Ontological Research produced Cannador, a standardized pharmaceutical preparation in the form of capsules containing cannabis grown in Switzerland and encapsulated in Germany. It agreed to provide the product free of charge. Researchers were concerned about ensuring continuous supplies of imported material: the use of Cannador depended on the ability of the charity to provide a continuous free supply, and the United States restricted THC production, which might limit its usefulness for large-scale clinical trials.[34]

Delivery systems were a major stumbling block. The clinical trials of THC in the 1970s and 1980s had been based on a capsule, but patients suffering from nausea found them difficult to take, and the effect of capsules had a long time lag in comparison with smoked cannabis. Smoked cannabis remained a pariah in an era of anti-smoking campaigns, though such trials were not ruled out. The protocols, however, eliminated smoking as a delivery method. Zajicek explained the decision for the CAMS trial: 'It was decided at an early stage that the drugs would be administered in capsules by mouth because of the increased dangers of smoking such drugs.'[35] The ultimate goal was a method of administration that provided the rapid absorption achieved by smoking. GW Pharmaceuticals hoped to solve the administration issue by producing a new delivery system for cannabis, but Zajicek had concerns: 'We knew from conversations with other companies that this was going to be quite difficult because it [a spray] is quite an irritant.'[36] As a result the CAMS trial went down the THC capsule route.

The trials faced numerous hurdles. In the United Kingdom a trial had to be approved by the MCA. Animal data would normally be expected from Phase I trials. Cannabis, however, was classed as a 'peculiar substance', and for once this worked in its favour. It had a long prehistory of use and of illicit self-medication within the community. Researchers hoped that the proof-of-principle trials

could begin with a cross between a Phase II and a Phase III trial.[37] The MCA initially wanted additional animal data, however, as
well as evidence on further aspects of the different cannabis extracts. This was a problem, as there were no facilities in Plymouth
for such work. A combination of events worked to the benefit of
the trials, as the issue was resolved pragmatically on the grounds
that GW Pharmaceuticals was to review animal studies, and widespread use of cannabis in the community made it unnecessary to
repeat the work.

Cannabis posed particular concerns for obtaining trial licences.
From the regulators' point of view there were major concerns over
the possible side effects. For example, the risk of psychotic effects
had always been an issue and was a particular worry in clinical
trials.[38] Though clinicians were aware of a potential risk, they cal-
culated that the difference between the medical dosage and the
recreational dosage mitigated the problem. Zajicek described the
implications: 'It's an increasing story that there is an association between psychosis and heavy illicit use. It's an association, and it may
not be causative but evidence is becoming more convincing ... You
can't shut your mind off to those issues but that is another reason to
do a long-term study ... In illicit use the amount ... is massive compared to licit medical use. You don't go out to get high ... you try to
lower the dose to avoid side effects.'[39] Regulators were concerned
over the extract arm of the trial, especially the CBD arm, because
CBD was less well known than THC. A compromise was reached: a
pilot study in Plymouth with a psychiatrist on standby.[40] No serious
problems emerged.

Other ethical concerns were common to all clinical trials. If a test
drug proved successful, and patients found it helpful, what were the
ethical implications of withdrawing a drug at the end of the trial
period?[41] In Zajicek's MS trial, a compromise was reached to place
patients back into treatment for an additional year. In the case of
the GW Pharmaceuticals trials, Guy emphasized that any patient who
believed that they had benefited during a study and who wished to
continue to receive material beyond the end of the trial would be
entered into a long-term safety extension. As Guy explained: 'This
is what politicians and ethics [committees] wanted.'[42]

Since cannabis was an illicit substance, support from the Department of Health and the Home Office was necessary for trials to take
place. Licences to possess any Schedule I drug for research had to
be granted by the Home Office on the basis that legitimate reasons

for research existed. To obtain a licence, researchers had to provide details of methodology and timescales, of ethical approval and safeguards for safe custody and record keeping, and of delivery methods that allowed for controlled dosages. Twenty-five licences for research projects on cannabis had been granted previously, and the Home Office stated that research was permissible under current mechanisms: 'Research into both cannabis and cannabinoids is possible within the existing policy and legal framework ... The Home Office and the MCA look sympathetically at ... research proposals and within the Department of Health we very much recognize the importance of research in this area and its potential value.'[43]

It was hoped that the provision of 'good practice' for trials would speed up the process of licensing, and licences were thus granted for the trials. Clinicians spoke highly of the assistance given by the Home Office in licensing trials after 1997. Zajicek described the facilitation: 'Everyone's been fantastic. When you do this kind of stuff you've got all these hurdles to overcome. The Home Office were great. The MRC was fantastic. It was relatively easy ... People were keen that it took place.'[44]

The necessity of importing the required drugs resulted in complications because international narcotics conventions required FDA export licences and Home Office import licences, and both had to coincide. This led to complicated logistics. It took time to coordinate, raising concerns over a long time lag for patients. The MRC-funded trials were not developed as a step towards licensing a CBM. If positive results were shown, a pharmaceutical company was expected to license a related drug instead. This would take time. GW Pharmaceuticals had produced a therapeutic preparation in order to license it should it prove successful in trials. But the hurdles that remained were no small matter: in order to see the provision of a licensed CBM, their product needed to pass successfully through the trials, and the drug then needed to proceed through the UK/ European regulatory system.

EMERGENT ISSUES OF THE CLINICAL TRIALS AND THEIR IMPACT

Both the proof-of-principle trials and the industry trials demonstrated few side effects and some benefits. But they also highlighted a number of emergent issues that were associated with clinical trials in general and others that were particular to the study of cannabis.

One of the main problems was recruitment. The first hurdle for the trials was to obtain the patient numbers that were required to run a large clinical trial: this was a necessity in order to overcome the criticisms about the evidence base resting on only small-scale studies. CANPOP aimed to investigate acute-pain relief following tonsillectomy or abdominal surgery,[45] but it suffered serious recruitment problems and was closed in October 2003 after only six patients had been recruited and randomized. The sample did not provide enough information to perform a statistical analysis.

Recruitment issues posed special problems for a study of cannabis, seemingly being subject to fluctuating public perceptions of cannabis's benefits versus its risks.[46] As Holdcroft complained later: 'Recruitment was so dependent on the media. If the media said something awful on recreational use, we didn't get people on the trial.'[47] Holdcroft commented on frequent media reports that linked cannabis use to mental health problems, and she recalled that 'lobbying from the psychiatrists emphasised the bad effects. It was this the media picked up on.'[48] At times the media presented an oversimplification of cannabis, which polarized a highly complex issue and distorted risk appraisals.[49] The perceived medical problems attributed to recreational use impinged on the clinical trials of therapeutic cannabis.

Clinicians found recruitment to be problematic for pain trials because there was a desire to recruit 'naive patients', i.e. patients who had not previously taken cannabis. Previous trials had focused on 'cannabis-aware' patients in order to overcome prescription problems, but this in turn had caused problems due to lay knowledge and the potential inability of the patient to cooperate in placebo-controlled trials. The discussions that had taken place with the MRC during protocol design meant that trials focused on the provision of the drug to 'naive' patients after surgery. It was deemed advantageous to utilize drug-naive patients because it provided better compliance with study requirements; however, such patients proved harder to recruit.

Retention posed further problems in the CANPOP trial because patients dropped out after surgery. Holdcroft described the problems with consent: 'The trial had significant technical problems ... [The MRC] said ... [cannabis] had to be assessed on its own without any other drug and with someone in moderate pain ... This led to ethical questions ... Should we not be using it along with the opiates? We had to take consent prior to someone entering [the] study ... In the cold light of day they could decide whether they wanted to be in moderate pain or not ... so we had to consent a large number of patients who never did the study as ... they could not take the oral medicine.'[50] The trial recruited pre-operation, but, when patients were in pain after surgery or were unable to take the capsules, many of them dropped out.

In pain treatment it was considered to be normal procedure to administer more than one drug, e.g. in combination with opiates. For licensing purposes, however, it was necessary to administer and measure only one drug: THC or an extract of cannabis. Holdcroft explained some of the problems that this approach engendered: 'Drug regulatory agencies only compare and consider a drug for licensing if used on its own ... If we use ibuprofen and morphine separately they do not provide as much pain relief ... they enhance each other's effect.'[51]

Holdcroft's initial patient in the familial Mediterranean fever trial discussed earlier used cannabis in order to reduce the amount of morphine that was required. In the later clinical trials researchers had to study cannabis in isolation. The trial design, which was created to suit regulations, therefore failed to trial one potential cannabis application, e.g. cannabis in combination with another painkiller.

When the CANPOP trial closed early in 2003, Holdcroft retained funding, which she intended to use to develop methodology for a new trial. But in the intervening period the medical environment changed. Technological advances in surgery reduced the intrusiveness of invasive surgery and the resultant pain. Furthermore, the failure of the first trial led to the MRC having concerns about funding another. Holdcroft commented on the MRC's decision: 'The money went back to the MRC. They thought it had taken too long and that perhaps it was not worth the money. We started with 4 hospitals. In the end we had over 20 ... so we had all these ready to start, then the MRC pulled the plug.'[52] The failure of the first trial and the loss of momentum weakened pressure for additional trials in acute pain, and interest swung towards chronic pain.[53]

However, trials in chronic pain posed other problems. Because of the regulatory process it was necessary to test a drug for chronic pain resulting from one disease: it could not be tested for chronic pain generally. This led to a guessing game over the choice of illness to test, not to mention the unknowns around long-term treatment for a chronic condition. Holdcroft explained the concerns: 'It has to be licensed for a certain sub-group of patients. It's like guessing who will benefit from it more. It can't be licensed for chronic pain; it has to be for a specific incidence, e.g. pain with stroke.'[54]

Nonetheless, interest in acute pain did yield some useful results, since a dose escalation section of the CANPOP trial was run successfully.[55] This investigation was a non-randomized dose-finding study to determine the dose of cannabis that was needed to achieve analgesia for post-operative pain within the main RCT. The study identified a dose of cannabis plant extract that could provide both pain relief and possible therapeutic benefit, and the trial researchers reported positive results on dosage in 2006.[56]

Issues of recruitment were less of a problem for the MS studies, but the time it took to recruit participants necessitated long-term projects. A subsequent trial on MS, known as CUPID (cannabinoid use in progressive inflammatory brain disease), took two years to recruit the full cohort of patients. The CAMS trial began in 2001 with 667 patients. Unlike the CANPOP trial, Zajicek found patients who were happy to take part in the CAMS trial and who were less scared off by adverse media reports.[57]

Retention in long-term trials for a progressive disease posed a particular set of problems. As Zajicek noted: 'It remains difficult to keep people on studies if they think they are getting worse, even if [we] think the line [of progression] is less worse.'[58] This led the clinicians on the CAMS trial to improve the measurement instruments in order to obtain statistically significant results in a shorter timescale. The new measures were also adopted for the follow-up CUPID trial.

A problem that clinical trials face in general is that patients often want to have the active drug, not the placebo. This posed a particular problem in the cannabis trials. Lay knowledge meant that patients were not 'blind': they soon became aware of which drug they received. Benchmark clinical trials were generally expected to be double-blind. It was unusual to test a new drug about which patients already possessed a good deal of knowledge and with which they may have been self-medicating. Patients were able to recognize the side effects of cannabis, and they tended to work out whether they were on the active drug or the placebo. It was possible for knowledgeable patients to take the drugs and to have them tested for the active ingredients. Zajicek recollected that 'one patient got the pills assayed for THC and found they were on the placebo. People knew what they were taking.'[59]

The problem was compounded because cannabis was readily available on the black market. Zajicek commented that it was 'more difficult to do long-term trials if there are other sources'.[60] This alternative source of available cannabis encouraged some patients to drop out of the programme. It also caused problems with gaining statistically significant results, and it opened the door to criticism over trial evidence in relation to a trial's validity. A major issue with any clinical trial is the placebo effect and unblinding, and the cannabis trials were no exception. Trials on cannabis were criticized on these grounds as well as on the grounds of efficacy. The MCA report on the GW trials highlighted some of the issues: 'The fact that a substantial proportion of patients had previously taken illicit cannabis as self-medication increases these concerns, firstly, because this may have enabled them to recognize Sativex by its psychoactivity, and secondly because they might have greater expectations of benefit from Sativex treatment than would cannabis naïve patients ... Differences from placebo on efficacy measures were small and there was concern that such differences could be accounted for by unblinding and measurement bias.'[61]

Patient knowledge led to patient selection issues and raised the concept of 'good patients'. CAMS clinicians found it important to select patients who were prepared to take part in a test, and they attempted to weed out patients who merely wanted access to cannabis. The problem had its humorous side; Zajicek commented on the selection of patients: 'Most clinical trials have dropouts – few trials [have] dropins ... It's about patient selection. It's important to choose people who do not behave badly.'[62]

The problems led some researchers to question the importance of the concept of unblinding in clinical trials. Zajicek argued that unblinding was not so important in the MS trial: 'If we can prevent patients becoming wheelchair-bound people aren't going to complain about some degree of unblinding.'[63] The MHRA accepted this compromise to a degree. In response to a similar problem in the GW trials, it commented that unblinding was not a major concern in the face of a compelling treatment.[64] The importance of unblinding appeared to be related to the efficacy of cannabis-based drugs, but proving efficacy was the biggest stumbling block for the trials and for the remedicalization of cannabis. Steering cannabis through clinical trials was one thing, but proving it was a valuable treatment for MS and pain was quite another. The CAMS trial, for example, reported a very small improvement in scores for all three treatment groups, and these improvements were slightly greater in the cannabis groups than the placebo group. None of these changes reached statistical significance, however. Results were published in *The Lancet* in 2003, and the CAMS study was criticized for similar reasons to the GW trials, including unblinding, the placebo effect, and efficacy.[65] But was it cannabis that was not efficacious or was it the clinical trials that were not able to accurately measure cannabis's effect?

Efficacy proved difficult to demonstrate, which was partly due to the outcome measures and the instruments used to test them as specified in the protocols. This was compounded by the nature of the disease under study. Holdcroft summed up the problem as follows: 'MS has been seen as the most acceptable disease in the United Kingdom for trials of cannabinoids. Unfortunately, there are probably few diseases that are harder to conduct clinical trials on.'[66]

The choice of disease under test was a problem, because the symptoms proved difficult to measure. A predetermined outcome measure is specified in a trial protocol and is expected to provide an objective measurement – it is an instrument against which success or failure is measured. A major hindrance to these trials was the problematic outcome measures that existed for MS and pain. A point in favour of using cannabis for MS was the fact that MS had a raft of symptoms, and cannabis might have a raft of impacts on the body. Robson explained the impact of cannabis's properties:

> One of the great strengths of cannabis is its breadth of
> effect against a range of symptoms ... In the beginning we
> tried ... to demonstrate that breadth of effect as one of the
> major assets of the drugs ... Unfortunately, the more you
> spread your target in a clinical trial the harder it is to get a
> statistically significant result. Also, because of the standard
> way of doing things in regulatory authorities ... they are
> looking for specific indications of drugs ... the nearer
> you can get to a magic bullet the better. Cannabis is not
> a magic bullet. That breadth of effect which is so valued
> by patients with multi-symptom disease such as multiple
> sclerosis or HIV/AIDS has been a handicap in getting it
> through the trials.[67]

This breadth of effect was one of the reasons why Paton had been wary of cannabis as a therapeutic as opposed to its use as a lead.

The lack of subtle outcome measures may have contributed to the failure to prove cannabis's usefulness to the extent required by clinical trials. Both the GW Pharmaceuticals and Zajicek trials used the Ashworth scale for measuring spasticity. This was a widely used scale because it was relatively simple and it aided reproducibility in experiments. The trials cast doubt on the measure's usefulness, however. As Zajicek later commented: 'Measurement methods are not subject to scrutiny or if they have been they have fallen below acceptable levels ... If we had a decent symptom measure for example in cannabis, they would probably all be licensed.'[68] The scale lacked sensitivity, especially over a short time span. Zajicek elaborated further on the lack of sensitivity of instruments that were available for the initial trials: 'The problem is that particularly in progressive disease we don't have the measurement instruments that reliably detect potential small levels of change, but levels that might be important to individuals ... There needs to be huge improvement.'[69] This in turn impacted on recruitment and retention. As Zajicek explained: 'The standard measurement is an awful measure. In order to see change you need three years ... deteriorating people don't want to stay in the study.'[70]

The patient perspective, however, showed that the trials were more successful than the outcome measures indicated. From listening to the patients, clinicians hoped that they were onto something, despite ambivalent results that were unsatisfactory to regulators. Zajicek recalled the disparity between the results and the patient experiences: 'Patients were rating that they found significant effects ... The bottom line was the primary outcome measures ... That study was not regarded as sufficient proof to use or license. We were left there with patients believing that the drug worked.'[71]

The dichotomy between the patient experience and the results as demonstrated by the outcome measures caused clinicians to extend the trial for a further twelve months, and this trial extension brought some of the first statistically significant results. These results also corresponded with new developments that had emerged from the laboratory in the 1990s on the role of cannabinoids in neuroprotection: 'Patients were followed up from the CAMS study for 12 months ... After 12 months we started to see positive results in the Ashworth score and another outcome measure of disability ... [the] Rivermead mobility index ... Over a year, we saw a spreading out of symptom benefit to other symptoms, like fatigue. To me this was very exciting but people took it with a pinch of salt.'[72]

The results from the trial extension were seen as sufficiently promising to warrant a further trial on a new application of CBM: one
that hoped to overcome earlier criticisms by making trials longer
and by incorporating new ways of measuring symptoms. Clinicians
aimed not only to show symptom relief but also to demonstrate the
exciting possibility that THC might slow the development of disability in MS. To this end a new trial called CUPID was developed. It
was funded by the MRC, which provided £1.5 million, with another
£1.5 million provided through a mixture of funding from the Plymouth Medical School, the MS Society, and the MS Trust.[73]

The supply of cannabis-based products for the trials was an ongoing problem. The reliance on a free, industrial source of synthetic
THC initially posed problems for the continuation of the CAMS trial
and then for the CUPID trial, with acquisitions and mergers disrupt-
ing the supply of Marinol. Unimed, which had supplied the THC for
the initial MRC trials, was bought out by the pharmaceutical firm
Solvay in 1999. It appears that Solvay may not have been aware of
the agreement with Unimed when they bought the company.[74] After
discussions with the clinical trials team, Solvay and the MRC turned
what had been a gentleman's agreement into a firm contract, in order to secure long-term supply.[75]

Solvay provided further funding to increase the monitoring of
the CAMS trial, in case it proved possible to move to licensing if there
was a successful outcome. According to Holdcroft, 'MRC trials tend
to be proof of principle and the science level of monitoring [is] less
than in industrial [trials]'.[76] Due to the ambivalent CAMS trial results, however, Solvay lost interest and did not supply THC for the
CUPID trial. They were more interested in a small study that was related to migraines than with the complexities of MS.[77]

At this point, George Cattier, a Solvay employee who had previously worked for Unimed, set up his own company, Insys. He
agreed to provide the THC free of charge, and he increased monitoring in the hope of moving towards licensing if trials proved
to be successful. Contracts were drawn up more tightly this time,
with the aid of the MHRA. The supply of cannabis extracts was less
complicated. The European Centre for Immunological and Ontological Research, which had undergone a name change to IKF
Berlin, agreed to continue supply, and they set up their own separate and substantial UK-based commercial trials on the relief of
MS symptoms.

New methodologies were developed. Zajicek and others began work on outcome measures, and they borrowed methodologies from the social sciences, including patient questionnaires. Other new technological developments were brought into the trials. In CUPID a host of other measurements, including scanning and a new spasticity scale, were added to the trial protocol. The new scale aimed to split the concept of spasticity into separate entities, including symptoms, psychological effects, and the effect on movement and mobility.[78] Zajicek argued that the trial was important for its methodological breakthroughs: 'Even if the drug does not work it will be a really important study in terms of the methodology ... We will be able to look at which bits of the measurement instruments are effective.'[79]

The GW Pharmaceuticals trials had been designed with the aim of bringing a drug to market. Phase I clinical trials began in late 1999 and proceeded to Phase III in 2001; these were carried out on patients with MS and neuropathic pain, and then in 2002 trials were carried out on patients with pain associated with cancer. The proof-of-principle trials had concentrated on THC in the form of Marinol, which was already licensed for another application. The process of making Marinol available for MS and pain would be relatively simple if efficacy was proven. However, GW attempted to license Sativex, a CBME, so the route to licensing was different and more complex than for a new chemical entity (NCE).[80]

The form of cannabis used in Sativex caused concern for the regulators. As discussed in the previous chapter, the House of Lords committee of 2001 questioned whether the MCA was biased over this cannabis-based drug and called into question their judgement:

> The MCA's decision to insist on further toxicology data on CBD could delay the production of a cannabis-based medicine by GW Pharmaceuticals by as much as 2 to 3 years. Were the MCA not to require further extensive toxicological studies on CBD, GW Pharmaceuticals claim that they could have a cannabis-based prescription medicine available for patients in 2003. We note that, according to GW Pharmaceuticals, the Canadian regulatory authorities have stated that they do not require additional animal toxicology studies for CBD. We put this to the MCA, who refused to comment. We found this refusal highly unsatisfactory.[81]

The problem was that GW Pharmaceuticals and the House of
Lords committee argued that cannabis extracts should not be considered as a new medicine, whereas the MCA was inclined to do just
that. Furthermore, the House of Lords committee argued that the
MCA was not treating cannabis in the same manner as other potential medicines and was placing undue emphasis on assuring safety
to the detriment of providing a remedy for patients. The MCA denied any bias.

In the meantime, pressure had been building for the rescheduling of cannabis, and, following expert committee reports in the
early 2000s, MPs voted to downgrade cannabis and its derivatives to
class C in October 2003, though cannabis possession remained an
arrestable offence as the power of arrest extended to class C drugs.
The reasons that were given for this alteration included a more accurate assessment of the harm caused by cannabis relative to other
drugs, the continued need to control cannabis use, and a signal that
the government wished to focus on the misuse of the most harmful class A drugs, such as heroin and cocaine. It marked a change
in the allocation of scarce resources from the control of 'soft' drugs
to 'hard' drugs. Debates in the House of Lords featured the consideration of the relative harms of cannabis compared with licit drugs,
with Lord Rea stating that: 'Although cannabis can precipitate some
mental illness it causes nothing like as much harm as alcohol or tobacco. Alcohol can kill people acutely – if they drink a whole bottle
of spirits – quite apart from causing lingering death and we all know
what tobacco can do in the long term. Those two substances are not
class A, class B, or class C – they are not classified at all.'

But despite this policy shift, GW struggled to move Sativex through
the licensing process. In 2003 GW submitted its licensing application, or 'marketing authorization application', to the MHRA. In 2004
the MHRA decided not to license Sativex in the United Kingdom because the Committee on Safety of Medicines was not satisfied with
the efficacy of Sativex in the indication sought by the company, stating: 'In reaching its advice the Medicines Commission ... considered
all the scientific data and arguments presented, and concluded that
the evidence of efficacy was insufficient to support granting marketing authorisations.'[82] Sativex was rejected not on the grounds of
safety but on the grounds of failure to detect useful effects. The
committee were concerned about the small-scale nature of the trials in comparison with most other commercial clinical trials, about

whether the trials were adequately blind, and about whether the trials showed any statistically significant effect.[83]

The patient community greeted the refusal of Sativex in the United Kingdom with disappointment. Commenting on the MHRA's decision not to grant a licence, Mike O'Donovan, the chief executive of the MS Society, expressed the belief that there was enough evidence that Sativex could alleviate spasticity.[84] The patient perspective appeared to be sidelined by the outcome measures, on which the decision was based. O'Donovan placed pressure on the Medicines Commission, which advised the MHRA, to be more flexible, emphasizing patient relief.

Nor did the proof-of-principle trials produce the results that activists had hoped for. The outcomes were inconclusive, and they failed to produce the evidence-based proof sought by the clinicians – even as the majority of patients taking part appeared to find benefits to their lifestyles. The problem partly centred on the method of administration, which, from the patient perspective, was an inferior model. Dr Layward later suggested that there were problems with the design of the trials from the start: 'The protocols got compromised so much. What you would like to do is often what you can't do in patients.'[85] Unusually, patients had practical experience of alternative methods. As it was not possible to test these, investigations took place on more 'acceptable' delivery methods, such as tablets containing cannabinoids, but from the patient perspective these lacked the effectiveness of smoked cannabis.

Patient associations questioned the nature of the evidence and the role of the patient perspective within the clinical trials assessment when results were published in 2003.[86] Researchers found that cannabis had no significant effect on the key symptom measurement of muscle spasticity as measured by the Ashworth scale. But the MS Society raised concerns about how patient perspectives were weighed as evidence, and it argued that a small statistical value in a test could have a significant impact on a patient's experience. It was difficult to quantify how a patient 'may feel' or to explain how 'more people on the drugs found relief from other very distressing symptoms like pain, spasm and sleeping problems than those taking a placebo'.[87]

The MS Society brought this perspective to the notice of medical advisory bodies. Along with other stakeholders, including manufacturers and health professionals' organizations, the society made submissions to NICE, the independent organization responsible for providing national guidance on both the promotion of good health and the prevention and treatment of ill health through health technologies. The society urged NICE to look beyond standard protocols and to think in more complex terms about the data. They insisted that the data may be 'muddied' by the variability in people's experience of MS symptoms and by the normal variation in people's response to cannabinoids. The society stressed that it was vital to 'take full account of the views of people affected by MS' – or, in other words, to 'walk in their shoes'.

The society pushed the legality issue and argued that the production of a legal medicine would provide a clear split between recreational and medicinal use, removing the risk of self-treating patients becoming entangled in the criminal justice system. Legal medical cannabis would limit 'distress and fear'. People would no longer have to choose between 'their health, personal safety, and careers'.[88] In short, the society's submission pointed to the wider context of the discussions about cannabis and the reasons why its potential as a useful medicine for those with MS was not being more squarely acknowledged in policy circles: 'People with MS are concerned that the political issues around recreational use of cannabis may unfairly influence a decision about cannabinoid-based medicines.' They claimed stigma was involved, whereas 'if a plant was discovered in the rainforest, then [it] probably would be called a miracle cure you know. It wouldn't have all this political baggage behind it.'[89]

FROM TRIALS TO LICENSING

The trials resulted in the first licensing of a cannabis-based drug based on extracts of cannabis in April 2005, when GW received regulatory approval for Sativex from Health Canada for the symptomatic relief of neuropathic pain in MS. This was later extended to adjunctive analgesic treatment in patients with advanced cancer. Iverson stated: 'The results with Sativex are clearly an important advance in the modern clinical development of a cannabis-based medicine.'[90] Regulatory approval encouraged big pharma, in the form of Bayer (later Bayer HealthCare), to enter into a strategic alliance with GW. Marketing this new drug was critical. GW announced that exclusive commercialization rights for the drug in the United Kingdom were licensed to Bayer AG and it provided Bayer with an option to expand their licence to include the EU and other world markets.

The licensing process proved more difficult in the United Kingdom, however. In 2005 GW Pharmaceuticals unsuccessfully appealed against the advice given by the Committee on Safety of Medicines to the MHRA, but the MHRA agreed with the Committee and requested further clinical efficacy data.[91] However, a system existed in the United Kingdom whereby drugs could be exempted from the licensing system and could be prescribed on a named-patient basis. Although Sativex was not licensed in the United Kingdom, it was issued to patients who had been in trials on a compassionate basis. After Sativex was licensed in Canada, and under pressure from both patients and doctors, the Home Office and the MHRA allowed the import of Sativex as an unlicensed medicine to be supplied on an individual-patient basis for MS under doctors' responsibility.[92] A press release from 2005 reads: 'GW announces that it has been informed by the Home Office that the Drugs minister, Paul Goggins, has confirmed that Sativex® oromucosal spray, its cannabis-based medicine, may be imported from Canada to satisfy its prescription to individual patients in the United Kingdom as an unlicensed medicine. This development is in response to enquiries from a number of UK doctors and individual patients who have been in contact with the Home Office to request access to Sativex.'[93]

The named-patient basis was a system used to provide off-licence drugs to particular patients and was most commonly used in oncology. This situation brought additional meaning to cannabis's borderline position: not quite approved, but sufficiently approved to permit its importation for use on a named-patient basis. Professor Holdcroft summed up the resultant situation: 'What I'm not sure is why the legal side hasn't changed for medical cannabis. Guy used a wedge through ... the named-patient basis. But it [Sativex] is quite expensive, not used everyday.'[94]

The Home Office granted GW Pharmaceuticals a licence that permitted the company to import a product that contained a substance that was controlled under the MDA. It did not consider lack of efficacy to be grounds to refuse importation, though the responsibility rested on the prescriber.[95] While Marinol had also been available on a named-patient basis, Sativex became more widely used and had been issued to more than 1,000 patients by 2006.[96]

In order to have the product licensed in Europe, GW Pharmaceuticals resubmitted its application for Sativex in 2006 via the European decentralized procedure of the European Agency for the Evaluation of Medicinal Products (European Medicines Agency (EMA) since 2007).[97] The procedure involved the United Kingdom acting as the reference member state, and if successful it would have allowed licensing across the EU. However, GW Pharmaceuticals withdrew the application before the end of the procedure in response to requests for further data. The MHRA provided regulatory guidelines to GW Pharmaceuticals for further work in order to help it succeed in another application.[98]

These procedures raised questions over the significance of the 'rule of evidence' and the role of clinical trials in licensing procedures. Professor Griffith Edwards summarized the dilemma as follows:

> I was wondering what the rules of evidence are ... I don't
> necessarily believe that controlled trials are everything and
> sometimes persuasive evidence of another kind is there
> before one's eyes ... There are also of course quite bogus
> claims made on single cases ... I deeply respect what our
> patients say and I wish doctors would listen more often
> and more closely. But I also know that medicine was once
> founded on what doctors believed and patients told and
> that really wasn't enough. We also need the evidence
> of science and to control the placebo effect. I am left
> puzzled that the controlled trials building on the brilliant
> laboratory work on endogenous cannabinoids etc., hasn't
> had its pinnacle in the application to clinical medicine ...
> I really would like to see more attention paid to the rules
> of evidence for our patients' sake.[99]

CONCLUSION

Clinical trials on cannabis emerged in the United Kingdom after a convergence of interests and scientific developments post-1995: lobbying from patients, developments in the laboratory, the interests of individual clinicians, the involvement of professional bodies, and the government's desire to split recreational use from medical benefits. These clinical trials had major impacts on the process of remedicalization. The trials that struggled to show effectiveness did indicate limited adverse effects and some potential benefits.

The trials also highlighted problems with clinical trial methodology – both issues generally associated with clinical trials and issues that were related to studying a drug that was based on a readily available illicit substance. Both the industry trials and the proof-of-principle trials brought extracts of cannabis into clinical trials for the first time in the United Kingdom. This was made possible by the emergence of standardized extracts and by a sufficient and regular supply and delivery of CBM. Trials began to move cannabis further through the process of remedicalization. In terms of legal provision of cannabis-based drugs, the industry trials resulted in one cannabis-based drug that was developed in the United Kingdom being licensed in Canada. This was the first cannabis-based drug to be licensed since dronabinol (Marinol) and nabilone (Cesamet) in the 1980s in the United States. This time the new drug was based on an extract rather than on synthetic THC.

Though no drug was licensed in the United Kingdom at this time, Sativex was made more widely available on a named-patient basis. In terms of methodology, the trials led to an acknowledgement of the limitation of available methods for the measurement of symptoms such as chronic pain, and they thus led to the development of improved patient-based outcome measures. This had the potential to lead to more successful outcomes of CBMs in future trials. The successful licensing of Sativex in Canada, and the proof-of-principle trials in the United Kingdom, extended the application of cannabis, beyond its anti-emetic properties, to MS and pain, and possibly towards neuro-protective aspects in the future. The development of clinical trials left various options open for licit CBMs, either through the development of existent synthetic products or through emergent cannabis-based extracts such as Sativex. After Sativex passed through the licensing system in 2005 in Canada, questions shifted to those around availability, cost, and access on the NHS.

8

Accessing Cannabis-Based
Medicinal Products, 2009–21

The 2009–21 period brings into stark relief many of the ongoing issues around cannabis that have been raised by this book: the interaction between medical and recreational use; the role of clinical trials; research–business links and the role of the pharmaceutical industry; supply; science–policy transfer and expert advice; and patient knowledge and advocacy. The use of a plant-based medicine continued to pose problems around the form of cannabis that was considered to be acceptable by different stakeholders. Cannabis, as a borderline substance, was still a conundrum for policymakers and patients. Although the period after 2009 is outside the main focus of the book, it is worth reflecting on the key developments of this period as they represent a continuation of unresolved issues that were discussed in the previous chapters.

This chapter looks at the rapid policy fluctuations that took place from 2009. After the mixed results of the clinical trials, cannabis's continued borderline status created a backlash. The trials did not provide a definitive answer: uncertainty over efficacy remained. While licit CBMPs were being researched and developed, licensed, and marketed, the attitudes of some scientists and policymakers towards cannabis appeared to be hardening again, resulting in cannabis being rapidly transferred back to the more restrictive Schedules in 2009. This left us with a paradox: while the United Kingdom was a pioneer in medicinal cannabis, becoming the biggest exporter of CBMPs by 2019,[1] few UK patients had access to these medicines. This led to a re-emergence of patient pressure, as both patients and researchers argued that regulation hindered access. This chapter looks at the reasons for this paradox.

Internationally, the appetite for CBMPs and cannabis seemed to be building, providing a shifting international backdrop to the UK debate. At the time of writing, across the globe remedicalization has produced various CBMs, ranging from botanical or herbal cannabis to synthetic single-entity tablets, mixtures of extracts of cannabis, and cannabis oil. This chapter sets the UK scene within the international context and discusses the provision of CBMPs that took place after the conclusion of the clinical trials.

RESCHEDULING CANNABIS FROM CLASS C TO CLASS B

This period highlights the continual debates between government, the pharmaceutical industry, researchers (especially in mental health), and patients. The legal frameworks governing licit and illicit cannabis use in the United Kingdom came under scrutiny again by a succession of governments and health secretaries, and cannabis's borderline position resulted in another rapid shift between Schedules. Cannabis's downgrading to class C in 2004 turned out to be rather short-lived, and in 2009 it was rescheduled back to class B.

It is worth looking back a little to see the reasons for this shift. Disquiet over the harms of cannabis, especially over mental health, has been a feature of the cannabis story throughout, and just as the clinical trials discussed in the previous chapter were taking place this came to a head. Concerns flared over the dearth of research in the addiction field, and pressure built for a more cautious approach to cannabis.[2] Fears rose over a link between cannabis and psychosis, especially from within the discipline of psychiatry, and especially in light of the increasing availability of more potent varieties such as 'skunk'. Robin Murray, a psychiatry professor at the Institute of Psychiatry, London, drew attention to new evidence that heavy cannabis use appeared to be linked to serious mental illness.[3] The government also faced criticism at the international level, as the UNODC chief, Antonio Maria Costa, argued against policy reversals (such as the downgrading from class B to class C) and the message that they sent to young people, claiming that countries received the 'drug problems they deserved'. Additionally, he contended that it was a mistake to dismiss cannabis as a 'soft' drug – a view that attracted growing attention in some sections of the media.[4]

In March 2005 the Labour Home Secretary Charles Clarke asked the ACMD to reconsider the scheduling of cannabis in light of this new evidence: the impact on mental health and the circulation of cannabis with a higher THC content. The ACMD, chaired by Michael Rawlins, recommended maintaining the status quo and argued against reclassification on the grounds that cannabis's harmfulness, either to the individual or to society, was not equivalent to the harmfulness of other class B substances.[5] The government accepted this advice, but the role of the ACMD was increasingly being questioned, highlighting flaws in the system of expert advice.

In 2006 the House of Lords Science and Technology Committee reviewed the relationship between scientific advice and evidence and the classification of illegal drugs as one of three case studies to inform its wider inquiry into the government's handling of scientific advice, risk, and evidence in policymaking.[6] The committee made fifty recommendations, of which the government accepted twenty-four and rejected twenty-six. The government rejected the suggestion that the ranking of drugs on the basis of harm should be decoupled from penalties. However, it agreed that the system was not fit for alcohol and tobacco.[7]

One of the most interesting aspects was the debate around the function of the ACMD. The House of Lords questioned both the operation and the composition of the committee, particularly the conflicting understandings of the ACMD's remit and the disagreements between its chair and the Home Secretary on classification. It was also concerned about the anomalies when classifying individual drugs, as well as the lack of consistency in the rationale for the classification of drugs. The government's response clearly showed that it was concerned that such criticisms might bring the integrity and independence of the ACMD into question. The government accepted that certain areas of operation could be improved: most notably transparency.

In relation to cannabis, the House of Lords questioned the timing of previous cannabis reviews, as they appeared to be a response to public outcry. The lack of public information that had accompanied the earlier reclassification of cannabis was heavily criticized. As we will see, questions of classification, the role of the ACMD, and the relationship between science and policy would plague future discussions.

The question of what to do with cannabis was not resolved, and the ACMD was again asked to reconsider the question in 2007. The ACMD made twenty-one recommendations and reiterated that cannabis should remain in class C.[8] This time the government was prepared to ignore the advice of its expert committee, and the Labour Home Secretary Jacqui Smith reclassified cannabis back up to class B in January 2009 on the grounds of more potent strains being available and the perceived threat to mental health. The reasoning behind this was not based on 'science' but rather on social and legal issues, as Smith stated that this decision took public perception into account: 'My decision takes into account issues such as public perception and the needs and consequences for policing priorities. There is a compelling case for us to act now rather than risk the future health of young people. Where there is a clear and serious problem, but doubt about the potential harm that will be caused, we must err on the side of caution and protect the public.'[9]

This provoked a series of public spats between the government and the ACMD, further highlighting the uneasy relationship between 'science' and policy that had been discussed in the House of Lords report. Professor David Nutt, a neuropsychopharmacologist, replaced Rawlins as chair of the ACMD in 2008 (he would go on to be the Edmond J. Safra Professor of Neuropsychopharmacology at Imperial College London from 2009). He clashed with the Labour Home Secretary Alan Johnson after writing an article on the perceptions of risk that compared ecstasy with horse riding in February 2009. Following the rejection of the ACMD report, Nutt accused ministers of 'devaluing and distorting' scientific evidence. Johnson expressed disappointment in Nutt's comments, but Nutt defended his response and the role of scientists in policymaking: 'If scientists are not allowed to engage in the debate then you devalue their contribution to policy-making.'

It appeared that science–policy transfer, always an uneasy relationship, was being brought into disrepute in a very public arena. In response, a group of scientists and advisers produced a statement on the principles for the treatment of independent scientific advice, which was backed by the then science minister Lord Drayson. Further problems emerged when Nutt delivered a paper at the Centre for Crime and Justice Studies, King's College London, arguing that illicit drugs should be classified according to evidence of harm, and that licit drugs such as alcohol and tobacco caused more harm than illicit drugs such as cannabis, LSD, and ecstasy. The Labour Home Secretary Alan Johnson then requested his resignation on 30 October 2009, declaring that his statements undermined the government's efforts to provide the public with clear messages about the dangers of drugs. Nutt resigned his position as chair of the ACMD. Richard Garside, director of the Centre for Crime and Justice Studies where Nutt had spoken, entered the fray, raising concerns about what this meant for the value of evidence-based policy: 'I'm shocked and dismayed that the Home Secretary appears to believe that political calculation trumps honest and informed scientific opinion. The message is that when it comes to the Home Office's relationship with the research community honest researchers should be seen but not heard ... The Home Secretary's action is a bad day for science and a bad day for the cause of evidence-informed policy-making.'[10] Five other members of the ACMD resigned in protest. Nutt continued to argue that the United Kingdom's increasingly hard stance on drugs was out of step with other countries that were softening their stance towards cannabis. Claims that there was an erosion of independence and political interference would dog the committee on and off for the next decade.

It is worth noting that by 2009 patients were also beginning to raise concerns around mental health. Patients largely appeared to give positive reports of Sativex, but uneasiness surfaced. Hodges, who had founded ACT, hinted that those suffering from MS were beginning to rethink the medicinal use of cannabis when she attended a witness seminar in 2009. She was unsure about Sativex and voiced concerns about the long-term effects of regular cannabis use on the mind, although she still found that it helped physically: 'I've become more ... aware of the downsides,' she recounted. She also noted the trade-offs involved: 'I can see that it's affecting my mind; not that it's making me psychotic, but I'm very conscious of it affecting my mind as well as helping my body.'[11] The debate over the link between cannabis and mental health continued throughout this period.[12]

UK POLICY IN THE CONTEXT OF INTERNATIONAL REGULATION

While the United Kingdom was tightening its control of cannabis, the extent to which medical cannabis was permitted in other countries varied enormously. Indeed, what we mean by medicalization and what is considered to be a medicine can vary in time and place.

Some countries, such as the United Kingdom, authorize only pharmaceutical grade medicines such as Sativex, while others permit controlled, standardized products, including cannabis oil: Canada and the Netherlands allow herbal or non-pharmaceutical preparations, for example. Access to CBMPs is provided via a variety of mechanisms: medicinal cannabis was legalized in Canada in 2000, while Uruguay legalized cannabis for recreational purposes in 2013. Canada moved one step further by amending 'medical access' to 'reasonable access' in 2016, and by 2018 it had legalized cannabis itself.

It should be noted that changes to the legal position do not necessarily improve access for patients. Canadian patients have highlighted that legalization has actually hindered medical access. Writing in *The Guardian* in 2020, Mike Power noted how suppliers shifted their focus from the medical market to the recreational market: 'In a stinging irony, medical patients – the very people whose decades of activism had driven the wider reforms, faced cannabis shortages and a steep increase in price after legalisation as suppliers diverted their medical product in bulk to the new recreational market rather than to smaller deals to medical patients.'[13]

By 2017 Sativex was approved in twenty-five countries around the world and was under investigation for potential indications of schizophrenia and other neurological conditions. Epidiolex/Epidyolex (CBD) became the first plant-derived CBM in the United States when it was approved by the FDA in 2018, and it gained approval by the EMA in 2019.

International agencies that had originally functioned as something of a countervailing force to remedicalization were softening their attitudes. As discussed earlier, the WHO had declared that cannabis had no medical value in 1952, but in 2018 the WHO's 41st Expert Committee on Drug Dependence (ECDD) recommended that cannabis and cannabis resin should be reclassified from their position alongside products that were deemed to be exceptionally harmful to the public, such as heroin. The committee noted that some cannabis-derived medicines – including cannabis extracts, tinctures, and preparations such as CBD – had no potential for abuse or dependence but did have significant health benefits for children with treatment-resistant epilepsy. It therefore recommended that they should be removed from international control regimes. The committee went on to scientifically review cannabis and other products derived from the cannabis plant, and in 2019 the WHO made a series of recommendations to the UN CND: to control cannabis preparations with high levels of delta-9-THC (dronabinol) more effectively but to allow further research and to improve access to cannabis-related medicines.[14] On 2 December 2020 the CND voted to delete cannabis and cannabis resin from Schedule IV of the 1961 Convention (they remain in Schedule I of the 1961 Convention). The CND decided not to follow the other recommendations made by the WHO.

The INCB, although wary of the medical cannabis movement, has stated that it does not prohibit medicinal cannabis provided that countries comply with the treaties.[15] One of the most significant developments came at the end of 2020 when the CND reclassified cannabis and cannabis resin under an international listing that recognized their medical value. Although the CND voted to accept the ECDD's primary recommendation on the reclassification of cannabis, it did not accept further recommendations made by the ECDD to change the classification of other cannabis-related substances, which the ECDD had hoped would improve their availability for medical use while at the same time preventing the harms associated with non-medical use.[16]

The prohibitive legislation of the 1970s had scared off most business interests, but the shifting attitudes of the international agencies in the twenty-first century led to resurrected interest from the pharmaceutical industry and the commercial sector. The medical cannabis market and the recreational cannabis market were increasingly seen as big business, involving multiple countries and companies exporting products and competing for market space. Global partnerships and a global market are adding a new dimension to the story.

UK PATIENTS MISSING OUT: WHAT GOVERNS POLICY AND PRACTICE?

Yet, despite these international moves, little had changed from the patient perspective in the United Kingdom. Chapter 5 discussed the influence that lay knowledge and activism had on the development of clinical trials and the form of cannabis that was used in the late 1990s and early 2000s. In this 2009–20 period, patient activism and the media again sought to influence policy and practice, as patient advocates brought medicinal cannabis back onto the political agenda, forcing changes to policy and regulation.

Patients contended that access to CBMPs was hindered by regulation and that they were only available for arbitrarily determined diseases. Significantly, the MS Society altered its long-held position in 2017 and called for the medicinal use of herbal cannabis to be legalized for MS patients. MS groups had been significant drivers of policy change in the United Kingdom in the 1990s because they were respectable patient groups that captured media attention, but by the 2000s new groups and diseases had become the driving forces behind policy change.

Between 2017 and 2019 there were heated discussions about patient access to cannabis-based drugs in relation to severe and rare forms of epilepsy in children. This was exemplified by the high-profile cases of two children, Alfie Dingley and Billy Caldwell, whose parents campaigned for access to cannabis oil, which they were able to obtain abroad but not in the United Kingdom. The children's plight garnered significant attention from the media, the public, and policymakers.

Alfie Dingley's parents had been told that the regular intake of steroids would eventually kill him, so they campaigned for access for cannabis. In the interim they obtained cannabis oil from the Dutch company Bedrocan. While they were living in the Netherlands, and under a paediatric neurologist's supervision, THC was added to the treatment plan. On their return to the United Kingdom, the parents pressed for access to a prescription for CBD and THC, but regulations made this difficult. Eventually, Mike Barnes, an honorary professor of neurological rehabilitation at Newcastle University, applied for and received the first UK licence for medical cannabis products. Dingley received medical cannabis oil in June 2018, and it was reported in the newspapers that he was 'amazingly well' after treatment.[17] Dingley's mother now leads a small campaign group called End Our Pain.

The Caldwell family travelled to Canada in 2018 to bring cannabis oil back to the United Kingdom, only to have it seized by customs on their return, resulting in Billy Caldwell being admitted to hospital four days later in June 2018. The Conservative Home Secretary Sajid Javid then responded and issued an emergency licence to allow medics to treat Caldwell with CBMPs. Rapid changes ensued after significant media attention and because MPs questioned access on behalf of their constituents. Javid called for a review on the grounds that the current state of play was unsatisfactory to all concerned. He stated: 'The position is not satisfactory. It's not satisfactory for the parents, it's not satisfactory for the doctors, and it's not satisfactory to me.'[18] In July of that year he announced plans to allow specialist doctors in the United Kingdom to legally prescribe cannabis-derived medicinal products. The Conservative Health Secretary Jeremy Hunt announced his support for the medical use of cannabis and indicated that another review would be undertaken to study possible changes to the law.[19] While the review was being carried out, an interim expert panel was created to advise ministers on any applications for licences.

The subsequent review consisted of two parts. One part was held by Dame Sally Davis, the Chief Medical Officer, on the evidence for the use of CBMPs. She concluded that there was conclusive evidence for the use of CBMPs for certain medical conditions, and she recommended that CBMPs be moved out of Schedule I. The second part of the review was carried out by the ACMD, which advised that cannabis-derived medicinal products 'of the appropriate medical standard' should not be subject to Schedule I. But here uncertainty over the definition of CBMPs was evident: with no standardized definition available, the ACMD required the development of a definition of CBMPs, and once products met the definition they would be rescheduled. CBMPs were subsequently defined as follows: 'Products must satisfy three conditions to be defined as "cannabis-based product for medicinal use in humans": a) is or contains cannabis, cannabis resin, cannabinol, or a cannabinol derivative (not being dronabinol or its stereoisomers); b) is produced for medicinal use in humans; and c) is— (i) a medicinal product, or (ii) a substance or preparation for use as an ingredient of, or in the production of an ingredient of, a medicinal product.'

While this was a significant move, it was also a limited one. Javid announced that cannabis products would be made legal for patients with an 'exceptional clinical need', and that cannabis would be moved from a Schedule I classification to a Schedule II classification.[20] However, this by no means meant immediate access for all patients: these products were still, on the whole, unlicensed drugs. But it did allow the prescription of CBM in certain circumstances via doctors on the General Medical Council's special register. This mechanism allowed the provision of 'specials' to cater for unmet medical needs. It meant that doctors would largely be prescribing unlicensed products, since at this time only Sativex had a marketing authorization (licence) in the United Kingdom, but as it was not viewed as cost effective it was not available on the NHS. The ACMD recommended that Epidyolex be placed in Schedule 5 to the 2001 Regulations. This was because THC is present only as an impurity and because it has a low risk of abuse potential, a low risk of dependency, and a low risk of diversion. Epidyolex (pharmaceutical grade CBD) from the United States went on to receive a marketing authorization from the EMA in September 2019, which meant that it became licensed in the United Kingdom.

CBD, which is not psychoactive, was not controlled under the MDA. However, due to the difficulties of isolating pure CBD, it could fall under the control mechanisms if it contained some THC (more than 1 per cent) as THC was a controlled substance. CBD has been designated a 'novel food product' under EU law (meaning that there was no long-term consumption prior to 1997), and readers might have seen it offered alongside their morning coffee or as part of the health and well-being market. Restrictions are tightening and it now needs a novel food authorization, which may impact on access to it in the EU and the United Kingdom.

These new provisions on CBMPs and 'specials' came into effect on 1 November 2018,[21] and Dingley received his prescription on 7 November. But because few CBMPs were licensed by the MHRA and approved by NICE, few were prescribed. The result was that clinicians remained concerned about prescribing CBMPs 'off licence', with limited 'evidence' to balance benefits and harms. By evidence they meant at least one RCT.

Although a licence could be obtained from the Home Office to import prescribed CBMPs, this did not mean rapid access for patients, and it was possible for the licence to expire prior to supplying the CBMP. As of mid-February 2019, virtually no one was able to access medical cannabis.[22] Cannabis oil, for example, was not recommended for use by NICE. In August 2019 NICE decided not to approve its use for children with severe epilepsy on the NHS due to a lack of clinical evidence. A review by the NHS stated that more trials were needed but that children's experience should be taken into account. NICE also turned down Sativex due to cost. Campaigners were severely disappointed. Genevieve Edwards, the MS Society's director of external affairs, responded firmly, highlighting the adverse

effects of the high costs on the society's members and pleading with
the government and the pharmaceutical companies to lower costs:

> NICE's refusal to recommend cannabis for pain and muscle
> spasms, or to fund Sativex on the NHS, means thousands
> of people with MS will continue to be denied an effective
> treatment … MS is relentless, painful and disabling
> and yet not a single person with MS has benefited from
> medicinal cannabis being legalized nine months ago. The
> government and the companies behind Sativex need to
> make people with MS a priority. Together with NICE, they
> must get around the table immediately to make Sativex
> available. This depends on the manufacturers accepting
> a lower price for the medicine, as right now the cost is
> entirely unrealistic.[23]

Dingley's mother queried why, given the law had changed, access
was not forthcoming.[24] Legal measures were the next recourse,
and in 2019 the family of Billy Caldwell launched a legal challenge
against the NHS and the Department of Health in Northern Ireland
over access to his CBM.

That same year, faced with criticism over the poor communication
about what the new provision would mean in practice, the House of
Commons Health and Social Care Committee reported on medical
cannabis, highlighting the barriers to research. Not for the first time
it argued that the research base remained limited because clinical
trials were restricted under the previous scheduling, and that new
trials were urgent. The committee stated that it was 'deeply sympathetic' and pressed the government to stop confiscating prescribed
medicinal cannabis that had been obtained overseas under specialist supervision.[25] They noted the need to build a robust evidence base
to make clinical decisions. They also considered the debate around
what 'evidence' should be accepted to demonstrate efficacy and
safety. They recognized that RCTs still constituted the gold standard
of evidence and that these remained the only way to obtain a licence,
but others were starting to argue for potential alternatives to RCTs.

Clinical trials were taking place globally, and witnesses called on
the committee to take notice of these studies. For example, Professor
Mike Barnes noted: 'At the moment, there are 128 trials of cannabis
ongoing worldwide. We should not forget that other jurisdictions

– sensible jurisdictions, if I can use that word – Canada, Australia, Germany, and other European countries, such as Denmark, have introduced cannabis legislation and allowed doctors to prescribe, and they are prescribing with more freedom than we are here. I think we are a little bit obsessed with UK-based evidence. We need to take into account global evidence.'[26] Despite these arguments, UK clinical trials remained the priority, as clinicians felt that evidence was weak, especially around certain conditions; as before, though, trials remained restricted due to regulations and constituted expensive long-term projects. Alternative evidence was available in the form of observational studies, but these had significant shortcomings and received little attention.

Previous chapters have highlighted the important role played by the pharmaceutical industry, and the issue once again came to the fore in the House of Commons Health and Social Care Committee's report: 'Medical products are usually developed by industry as they stand to profit from investing in the research. However, in the case of medicinal cannabis, this is not happening in part because of the difficulty in obtaining patents for medicinal cannabis products. The call for research proposals by the National Institute for Health Research demonstrates that the public sector is taking the lead in this area but it is also important for industry to be more involved in developing medicinal cannabis products and supplying products for research.' Industry involvement was critical for supply. Indeed, the committee went so far as to demand it: 'The Department of Health and Social Care should investigate those instances where pharmaceutical companies do not provide their medicinal cannabis product for research and take appropriate action where necessary. The Department should not be afraid to "name and shame" companies who are not doing all they can to make their products available for research. The Department should also set out a plan to encourage industry to take a more active role in research itself and should present this plan in response to this report.' The spectre of Brexit was also a concern for the committee due to the potential disruption of collaboration across Europe, as well as a break in supply chains. However, the government argued in response that a legal route now existed to prescribe and supply CBPMs in the United Kingdom without recourse to treatment or supply from abroad.

Discussion also took place on managing high patient expectations about availability after rescheduling, but patients had been pointing out since the 1990s that they needed help during these time lags between clinical trials and access to a medicine, rather than leaving it to some indeterminate point in the future. Urgent questions were once again raised in parliament when more patients had their medicines confiscated on their return to the United Kingdom after travelling abroad to obtain medicine, and MPs again began asking questions on behalf of their constituents. The Conservative Health Secretary Matt Hancock, who had replaced Jeremy Hunt, sympathized but left the decisions to clinicians. The NHS was again asked to carry out a rapid process review. It concluded that the understanding of CBMPs was variable among clinicians, that the lack of RCT data was a barrier to prescribing, and that patient expectations following rescheduling were high. Ten recommendations were made, largely around improving information on the subject.[27]

In May 2019 Nutt complained about the barriers to access and argued for another route: namely, adopting the cancer research model, with small expert groups conducting open effectiveness studies (which are different from the efficacy sought in clinical trials, as these are a test in real-world situations) to collect data on outcomes and side effects.[28] Drug Science, an 'independent science body' founded by Nutt in 2010, announced that it would set up Europe's largest patient registry, aiming to improve patient access and to carry out research. It aimed to run a two-year trial (Project Twenty21) with 20,000 patients through a patient outcome registry in conjunction with the Royal College of Psychiatrists, the British Pain Society, and the United Patients Alliance, testing cannabis products for chronic pain, epilepsy, MS, and post-traumatic stress disorder. By teaming up with private clinics, the provision of CBMPs would include THC-only medications, CBD-only medications, and a combination of the two cannabinoids, available at a subsidized cost. Partnerships were formed, with one example being that with LYPHE, a patient access system that provides clinics, dispensing services, import infrastructure, and educational services to patients, doctors, and industry.

In November 2019 NICE changed its guidelines to consider CBMPs such as nabilone as treatments for intractable nausea and vomiting and to offer trials of THC:CBD for spasticity. No CBMP was offered for chronic pain and no recommendations were made for severe treatment-resistant epilepsy, though NICE made research recommendations. Some patients' groups called this a missed opportunity.

In response, the chair of the ACMD requested from the Minister of State for Crime, Policing and the Fire Service that Epidyolex should be moved to Schedule V, as it had a low risk of abuse, dependency, and diversion. This was accepted, and Epidyolex was fast-tracked and became available from January 2020. In March 2020 the Department of Health and Social Care and the Home Office made an announcement that import restrictions on 'specials' had been changed: companies were now allowed to import CBMPs in advance of a prescription, and in bulk, to ensure that patients' prescriptions were not delayed or interrupted. In continental Europe the first EU-wide marketing authorization for a cannabis-derived medicinal product was granted by the EMA to Epidyolex as a therapy for seizures.

New access mechanisms were also developed in the United Kingdom. Charlotte Caldwell, the mother of Billy, withdrew her legal challenge to acquire medicinal cannabis for him in September 2020. Instead, it was now possible for her to pursue access through the Refractory Epilepsy Specialist Clinical Advisory Service panel led by neurologists from Great Ormond Street Hospital in London. The National Institute for Health and Care Research (NIHR) had opened a call for primary clinical research into the safety and clinical effectiveness of CBMPs in 2018, but this closed in 2019 after attracting only one application, which was declined.[29] The NIHR will potentially carry out two large-scale clinical trials for epilepsy but they have not yet commenced. Clinical trials of Sativex continued for other applications.

Private prescription was another route to access, but this was not without its own problems. Carly Barton, one of the first patients to receive a private medical cannabis prescription after the law changed in 2018, was burdened with spiralling costs, so she sought additional solutions. She created Carly's Amnesty, which set the stage for Cancard, which was launched in November 2020. The card costs £19.99 per year plus a one-off £10 administration fee. It is targeted at people who qualify for a private prescription of medicinal cannabis but are unable to afford one so may seek to obtain cannabis illegally. It was hoped that the card would help the police exercise discretion in relation to cannabis possession from patients medicating for their condition.[30] It was designed with the help of doctors, backed by senior representatives of the Police Federation, and it also received the support of various MPs, including Crispin

Blunt, the head of the Conservative Drug Policy Reform Group. It was not without controversy, however. In 2021 the BMA and the Royal College of Physicians warned that they did not support the card: 'The Cancard UK website states that the Cancard has been designed in collaboration with GPs but as far as we are aware there is no formal endorsement from the Royal College of GPs, nor has the BMA, as your trade union, been consulted.'[31]

Cannabis, whether medical or recreational, is potentially lucrative. In 2020 the BMJ published an investigation into big business links and the increasingly blurred lines between medical and recreational uses; it also looked at the growing pressure to gain access to the potentially lucrative recreational market.[32] Murray, who had raised the issue of the link between cannabis and psychosis in 2020, voiced concerns about the influence of the 'wild west cannabis industry' in light of the experience of legalizing cannabis in Canada and in some US states: 'I didn't appreciate how big the cannabis industry was going to be. These guys in Canada and California, they are setting out that the cannabis industry will be as big as the tobacco industry.'[33] Limiting access to CBMPs has left an opening for other interests to fill the niche, while patients complain that legalization has in fact detracted from medical access.

I have previously shown how government concerns over recreational use had encouraged research into cannabis and the development of pharmaceutical-grade cannabis medicine as a way of splitting the medical and recreational spheres, allowing for medical cannabis to exist without encouraging recreational use. This approach appears to have faltered. The limited medical use of cannabis is increasingly resulting in networks between patients, industry, producers, and investors becoming a powerful influence on cannabis policy. The question is whether the failure to provide wider access to pharmaceutical-grade cannabis has opened the door to pressure for the legalization of recreational use.

Brexit adds yet another complication, highlighting the issues of supply that have long had an impact on the development of CBMPs. Just as families thought that the cannabis oil problem was on the way to being resolved, Brexit regulations threatened to hinder supply, as prescriptions were not included in the trade deal.[34] Most oil is imported from the Netherlands. It was reported that Alfie Dingley's mother was given two weeks' notice of the fact that, due to the end of the Brexit transition period, prescriptions that were issued in the United Kingdom could no longer be dispensed in EU member states.[35] How Brexit will impact both the UK medical cannabis market and patients remains to be seen.

CONCLUSION

The 2009–21 period highlights ongoing debates around cannabis and how it has remained something of a Catch-22 situation. Cannabis had been remedicalized to a certain extent by 2009–21 – multiple CBMPs had been developed, and the United Kingdom had become one of the world's biggest producers – but these products were not readily available in the United Kingdom, and patients were increasingly clamouring for access.

Almost fifty years after cannabis tincture was removed from the United Kingdom, questions remain unresolved over what governs policy and practice around cannabis and other borderline substances. This chapter has highlighted the continuing role of uncertainty; what constitutes evidence and who controls that evidence; the impact of frameworks governing licit and illicit cannabis use; and the role of patient groups. It has also illustrated the importance of terminology: what do different groups mean by CBM, and how does that vary for time and place? The chapter also brings forth an additional dimension that looks likely to be critical in decades to come: the expanding role of research–business–patient collaboration. Commercial interests across the globe are becoming very influential. Limited access to CMBPs means that, far from being split from recreational use, this stage of remedicalization is increasingly tied up with commercial interests and potential pressure from vested interests for a recreational cannabis market.

Conclusion

Cannabis is a complex substance, because of both its chemical structure and the baggage that it carries. Cannabis's position in society has been determined by different stakeholders at different times, with each claiming a different role for the plant. In the twentieth century cannabis constituted a headache for the regulators of both medical and illicit drugs. Its multifaceted and fluid role has meant that cannabis has proved difficult to classify definitively, and yet its relationship with other drugs, both medical and recreational, is important as its borderline position acts as a spotlight on drug policy. But how did we get from the WHO's 1952 pronouncement that cannabis had no medical value, and its removal as a medical substance in the United Kingdom in 1973, to the United Kingdom being one of the world's biggest exporters of medicinal cannabis? Furthermore, what did this journey mean for cannabis as a medicine and for its position in the drug control framework?

Cannabis's role as a medical substance never disappeared entirely. Its medical role was maintained by some within the patient community, and scientific research continued – albeit in a very limited manner – even when its dual structure was denied by policy. During the period under study many of the problems that had previously hindered cannabis's transformation from a drug to a medicine in the nineteenth and much of the twentieth century were overcome, facilitating remedicalization.

SCIENTIFIC KNOWLEDGE

Changing scientific knowledge contributed to a shifting environment around cannabis. Science had played a role in the post-war marginalization of tobacco, and it had played an important role in the remedicalization of cannabis as well. Medicinal chemists, pharmacologists, sociologists, psychiatrists, neurologists, and anaesthetists all contributed their expertise to the developing understanding of cannabis and to its application as a medicine. This took place within the context of the rise of more specialist disciplines, such as clinical pharmacology, psychopharmacology, and phytopharmacy. Personal and, later, professionalized scientific networks pulled disparate researchers together and stimulated breakthroughs, any one of which, if missed, might have stopped remedicalization.

Major discoveries – including the isolation of the active principle, THC, the synthesis of cannabinoids, and the discovery of the ECRS – reinvigorated the field at critical points. The discovery of the ECRS conferred legitimacy on anecdotal reports of cannabis's therapeutic use, e.g. it demonstrated the importance of this system in the modulation of pain and opened up new avenues for research. Advances in other fields, such as cloning, contributed to advances in understanding. In addition, technical developments, including mass spectrometry, enabled research to progress at a faster pace and allowed for more subtle analysis in experiments. But 'blue sky' research is rare, and individual and disciplinary interest was supplemented by the broader, twin needs of drug control and medical necessity.

Political and social fears over cannabis's recreational use and subsequent developments in drug control were paramount in the process of remedicalization. In the search for solutions to the drug problem, countries such as the United Kingdom pursued not a medical approach but a control-oriented one. There was a global dimension to this that was driven largely by the United States. Medical utility was critical for the placement of drugs within drug control legislation, and cannabis's role as a medicine was eroded at the policy level. Though international and domestic drug control systems acted as a countervailing force against medical uses of cannabis, they also provided a dual spur to remedicalization.

Drug control imperatives directed funding towards the cannabis field. Treating cannabis as an illicit drug created a need to improve the knowledge base for control purposes, pulling scarce resources into the cannabis arena. Though initial research focused on its deleterious effects, research indicated some medical applications during the process of understanding the pharmacology of cannabis. For example, Paton's work on cannabis's pharmacological relationship with anaesthetics indicated analgesic properties, an area that was investigated by clinicians in depth from the 1990s on-wards. When scientific research emerged on cannabis's applications as an anti-nausea agent and in the treatment of diseases such as glaucoma, asthma, and epilepsy, it began to overturn the viewpoint enshrined in policy that cannabis's medical use was obsolete.

But the question in the early 1970s was whether it was wise to uti-lize cannabis as a medical drug. In light of its potential harms and its potential as a drug of misuse, not to mention its pharmacological complexity, researchers like Paton answered that it was not. Never-theless, by the mid-1970s other pharmacologists were beginning to argue that it was wise to consider cannabis as a medical drug, and it appeared that cannabis's potential as a medicine had begun to out-weigh its possible harms. This was especially the case where there was a clear unmet medical need for high-profile medical problems, such as in the management of cancer treatment. As the cannabis story demonstrates, scientific knowledge and evidence is multifac-eted and ever-changing. Policy needs to be capable of adapting to changes that take place in the knowledge base, which, it should be noted, can vary across disciplines or even between scientists within the same discipline.

SCIENCE–POLICY TRANSFER

The transfer of science to policy was enabled by the development of a mechanism of expert advice via expert committees and by the desire to place policy on a stronger evidence base, especially in the field of illicit drugs. Cannabis's borderline position and wide-spread use within the community meant that considerable time was spent discussing the drug, and the initial expert committees in the 1970s and 1980s provided early discussions of cannabis's potential as a therapeutic.

The drug problem had been framed under the criminal justice sys-tem, but – as the limitations of this were revealed and other pressures mounted, from both the focus on civil liberties and the practicalities of implementing a penal approach – new approaches were sought. Early public reports, such as the Wootton Report, downplayed the harms of cannabis and raised the profile of the therapeutic use of derivatives of cannabis in policy circles and in the public domain. The closed discussions of the ACMD sub-committees also contributed to a shift in the policy environment. Because cannabis lost its dual structure, cannabis discussions inevitably had to cover emergent therapeutic indications. The use of cannabis by patients highlighted some of the problems of a penal response and necessitated evaluation of where responsibility for medical cannabis lay.

The United Kingdom had a more flexible attitude towards the medical use of controlled drugs than did the United States. In the United Kingdom, for instance, diamorphine (heroin synthesized from morphine) had legal pharmaceutical status when it did not in the United States. Under the British system there existed medical and non-medical structures for the drug. Opium also existed under both legal proscription and medical prescription, as its alkaloids, such as morphine, retained their duality.

Licit tobacco, on the other hand, moved further in the opposite direction: it had no medical value, and with the evidence of harms gradually being accepted, it became increasingly regulated as its cultural acceptability diminished. Cannabis, or at least its derivatives, retained the potential to return as a prescribed product and to regain its dual structure. In the meantime, research and the drug's emerging scientific legitimacy began to influence discussions on cannabis policy more generally. Whichever policy was to be adopted and implemented, scientific research was required.

Without this driving force to improve the knowledge base, cannabis might have remained a poorly understood herbal product. The policy structures around cannabis, including the ACMD, the Home Office, and the DHSS, all demonstrated shifts towards accepting cannabis as a medicine in some form. As cannabis began to regain medical credibility, policymakers saw the advantage to be gained by recreating the dual role for cannabis, as it offered the opportunity not only to split the medical use from the recreational use of cannabis but also to weaken demands for legalization in the process. The debates within the ACMD show how the scientific advice behind recommendations can be mixed, and the government's acceptance or rejection of any such advice demonstrates how advice may be adopted or rejected to suit contemporary political priorities.

INTERNATIONAL AGENCIES

The attitudes of international agencies towards CBMs underwent something of a change. Emergent therapeutic uses overturned the WHO's 1952 pronouncement that cannabis had no medical use, and by the 1990s the WHO began to take a softer line towards medical applications, e.g. its recommendation for dronabinol to be down-graded in the 1990s. Similarly, the INCB had to concede some limited medical utility by the 1990s, if perhaps only to retain its authority and the integrity of the drug control framework.

The stigma around cannabis was difficult to dispel, however, as evidenced by the divisions between the UN agencies over dronabinol's placement within the UN 1971 Convention on Psychotropic Substances. Furthermore, the acceptance of herbal cannabis or medical marijuana, as advocated in some US states and in Canada, was in no way accorded a similar shift in attitude. Cannabis was originally caught up in international legislation, and while this book has focused on the United Kingdom, it is really an international story – one for which the response of the international agencies has proved crucial. International development and international knowledge exchange is an integral part of the story. Any individual country's policy needs to be seen in the wider sphere, especially in relation to medical cannabis, as the pharmaceutical industry, commercial firms, and investment companies become involved and operate beyond country boundaries; this resulted in the paradox of there being limited UK patient access to cannabis despite the country being the world's biggest producer.

INDUSTRY

In transforming the concept of cannabis 'the drug' into cannabis 'the medicine', the pharmaceutical industry was fundamental. Industry development of CBMs appeared to offer a way of accepting cannabis's medical utility at the same time as transferring the ownership from 'illicit' drug users to the professional medical sphere by putting into place medical and regulatory structures around cannabis-based drugs.

In the nineteenth and early twentieth centuries, during the professionalization of medicine, patent medicines were sidelined and self-medication was attacked. Commercial products and treatments shifted away from the control of pharmacists and patients and towards pharmaceutical products that were regulated by the government. This avenue was deemed to be acceptable by policymakers and by the medical establishment, in contrast with patient attempts to self-medicate with unstandardized, herbal products.

The isolation of THC encouraged the interest of the pharmaceutical industry in the 1970s, which then provided the first licensed CBM since the removal of the tincture. Industry provided single-chemical-entity synthetic drugs – chemically manipulated versions of the main psychoactive phytocannabinoids. Some of these proved to have too many side effects and never made it to the clinic, but they re-stimulated academic research. Although the lack of industry–research links hindered supply in the 1970s, other cannabis-based drugs such as nabilone were tested in the clinic and made the leap through the regulatory process in the 1980s, though they did not reach a wide market. The drugs might have been introduced because of a focus on cancer – a high-profile and emotive disease – but due to the stigma of cannabis still being present, along with strict controls and the advent of additional drugs for these applications, industry soon lost interest.

The relative failure of the single-chemical-entity drugs left the door open for demands for herbal cannabis and the development of additional CBMs. In the 1990s the niche that was left open by synthetic CBM stood ready to be filled. Cannabis therapeutics benefited from the changing structure of the pharmaceutical industry. The development of biotechnology firms filling niche markets that had been neglected by big pharma allowed for a newly created small firm, GW Pharmaceuticals, to take an alternative route through the process of remedicalization: phytomedicine. To an extent, some of the constraints imposed on big pharma by the stigma around cannabis were not relevant to a scientist–entrepreneur who had belief and expertise in phytomedicine. As the remedicalization of cannabis demonstrated, the relationships – either via informal links or, today, more through formal partnerships – that are emerging between the pharmaceutical industry and other key stakeholders is pivotal for the process of drug development.

PHYTOMEDICINE

Phytomedicine – which had originally filled the medicine chest but had then been marginalized as the pharmaceutical industry developed and concentrated on synthetics – began a comeback in the late twentieth century. It provided a route to integrate user activists' demands for access to herbal cannabis while at the same time providing a standardized and regulated medicine.

The myriad of constituents found in cannabis, as in any plant, posed problems in early research, but in later years they looked to be a key benefit. The desire to create a medicine out of herbal cannabis led to heated debate over the form to be researched, developed, and licensed. Should it be cannabis, THC, or other cannabinoids, either singularly or in combination? My research has demonstrated a shift from the search for and development of single chemical entities, usually synthetics, to a re-emergence of interest in botanical cannabis. That change was facilitated by the rise of phytopharmacy and the biotechnology industry.

Close relationships between industry, academia, and the government proved decisive in the 1990s, as evidenced by the story of GW Pharmaceuticals. The government licensed GW to develop CBMs, and GW offered the long-sought-after domestic supply. It was able to solve another of the key problems that had plagued cannabis: standardization of the raw material on an industrial scale. GW's focus on a botanical substance – a traditional medicine (not an NCE) – meant that a product could be brought relatively quickly to market. This was advantageous when there was so much pressure to make cannabis available as a medicine. The relationship with big pharma was important. By the early twenty-first century, big pharma was showing an interest in phytomedicine, and a strategic alliance was formed between Bayer AG and GW that enabled Bayer AG to market licensed Sativex medicines.

The debates over form were important for the process of remedicalization as they impacted attempts to draw a distinct line between recreational and medical use. Cannabis was a borderline substance, but it was its derivatives that had more potential to be treated more flexibly. Once CBMEs were introduced, it could be argued that there was no further requirement for the use of herbal cannabis, which was more likely to remain static within the drug control framework. The remedicalization of cannabis demonstrates that the ways in which we view and investigate plants and their constituent parts are important for the development and the licensing of medicines. This includes how we incorporate traditional or lay knowledge, who has ownership of intellectual knowledge or 'evidence', and how plant-based medicines fit into the existing clinical trial system.

DELIVERY SYSTEMS

The ability to deliver cannabis via a new delivery system was another factor in its remedicalization. In the 1970s Paton had queried if the method of delivery was the best means of controlling the drug.

Nineteenth-century technological developments in drug administration systems had helped to marginalize cannabis, as it is not water soluble and thus was not suitable for the new hypodermic syringe. While the development of synthetic single-chemical-entity cannabinoids delivered via tablets was acceptable to policymakers and to the pharmaceutical industry, it proved less acceptable to patients, who maintained a preference for smoked herbal cannabis. In the 1990s GW's new delivery system, an oral-mucosal spray, offered a number of advantages. It avoided smoked cannabis, a no-go for policymakers and the medical community; it provided a measured dose; and it bypassed the problems associated with oral administration that had beset the single-chemical-entity drugs, providing patients with something more akin to the advantages of smoked cannabis.

EXPERT ADVICE: PROFESSIONAL BODIES

Cannabis therapeutics in the United Kingdom would not have advanced as it did after the 1990s without the legitimacy conferred on the concept by influential professional bodies such as the RPS and the BMA. When the BMA produced a reasonably favourable report on cannabis therapeutics in 1997, it boosted cannabis's legitimacy. This was important in the context of the influence of the medical profession and the close relationship between the state and medicine. The RPS provided the practical framework on which to build the recommendations of the BMA report, and it brought researchers, industry, funders, and policymakers together with a single aim: to carry out clinical trials on cannabis that would hopefully lead to a CBM. The House of Lords Science and Technology Committee also brought together all the stakeholders in an open forum, helped to alter the policy environment around cannabis, and, most importantly, provided the momentum to turn the concept of medical cannabis into a reality.

LAY KNOWLEDGE

The incentive to study cannabis as a medicine would not have been so great without the role of lay knowledge. Cannabis's position as a botanical substance was important, as it meant that the general public had access to and intellectual knowledge of the drug in advance of it becoming a pharmaceutically produced product, in contrast to most other medicines. Despite increased controls on drugs, there remained widespread illicit access to cannabis, so a battle over the 'ownership' of cannabis emerged.

Lay knowledge of cannabis drew attention to its medical properties for a raft of problems, including its use as a palliative in the 1970s; for treating glaucoma; for AIDS in the 1990s; and also for MS and pain. Thus, knowledge of cannabis's therapeutic qualities combined with the illegal status of cannabis led to the development of lay advocacy. Although medical arguments emerged as a component of 1960s legalization activism, in the United Kingdom medical activism for research and access to cannabis for MS became particularly important in the 1990s. High-profile advocacy combined with high-profile legalization demands that developed in this period placed pressure on policy. The result was the facilitation of clinical trials and an incentive for the pharmaceutical industry, in the form of GW Pharmaceuticals, to risk the costs of research and development because of the acknowledgement by the government that if an evidence-based drug could pass through clinical trials it could be licensed in the United Kingdom.

Lay knowledge and advocacy was also critical in focusing the direction of research. This included the form of cannabis to be studied, making research into extracts of cannabis imperative. It was important for forcing researchers, industry, and regulators to take account of the patient perspective – no small point in medicine. Patient experience also forced researchers to re-evaluate outcome measures in clinical trials. Finally, when no drug was forthcoming after the development of trials, patient concerns contributed to the circumvention of the regulatory system through the import of Sativex – on a named-patient basis and as a temporary measure – and, in more recent years, those concerns have also led to the fast-tracking of Epidyolex. Patients wanted these new drugs on the NHS but, with minimal provision, the need was increasingly fed by private prescriptions. Patients either resorted to expensive purchase of the medicines or illegal access to cannabis.

Patient knowledge and patient voices are too often dismissed, yet, as shown by the cannabis story, they can have an important role to play in the development of medicine, especially for symptoms that can be very subjective, such as pain. A recent example is patients being important in having loss of taste and smell added to the Covid-19 symptoms list. How we integrate the patient voice into medicine requires further study.

CLINICAL TRIALS

As these driving forces coalesced, they resulted in a concerted effort
to place cannabis in the clinical trial system, providing the opportunity to prove cannabis's safety, efficacy, and quality, as demanded
by the MHRA under the Medicines Control Act of 1968. The trials
that took place demonstrated safety if not efficacy, and the issue
of the latter, it was argued, could be related not to cannabis but to
the very methodology of randomized clinical trials themselves. The
study of plant-based products, especially for the treatment of subjective issues such as pain, highlighted the inherent problems with the
methodology of RCTs and the regulatory mechanisms. By 2017, however, Sativex had been approved in twenty-five countries around the
world and was under development for potential indications of schizophrenia and other neurological conditions. The remedicalization
of cannabis highlights the importance of clinical trials. Clinical trials are viewed as the gold standard of what may be thought of as
constituting evidence, but remedicalization also raises questions
over how we use them, their methodology, their results, and their
interpretation, as well as how they fit with other forms of 'evidence'.

*

In summary, the United Kingdom had been a pioneer in the pharmacology of cannabis, and it was a UK pharmaceutical company
that developed a cannabis-based extract and enabled the United
Kingdom to become the world's biggest supplier of medicinal cannabis. But while trials in the United Kingdom and the licensing of
Sativex represented another step in the process of remedicalization,
there remains a wide gap between product development and provision to patients, and demands for patient access have unsurprisingly
dominated discourse within the United Kingdom since 2017.

Just as the clinical trials did not end the medical utility argument,
nor did they mark the end of the debate about cannabis's position
in the drug control mechanisms. Uncertainty has been a recurring
feature in the story of the process of remedicalization. Throughout
the period under study, uncertainty around medical efficacy and
possible harms has enabled politicians to interpret the 'science'
and to pursue their own agendas. As a borderline drug, the rapid
fluctuations of cannabis's position drew attention to the validity or

otherwise of the control system. Cannabis remained a 'dangerous medicine', and cannabis harms included its threat to the stability or the structure of the control framework. There were calls for the entire system to be re-evaluated, and comparisons were drawn between cannabis and licit drugs, such as alcohol and tobacco. The subsequent disagreements between the government and the ACMD highlight issues around science–policy transfer, the role and the limitations of expert advice, as well as evidence-based policy and transparency in the decision-making process.

Writers have shown how little history has spoken about policy in the drug control field, and they have complained about the selective use of history in the field's formation. A knowledge of the history of drug control policies and the substances that these policies control is important for future policy around illicit drugs and medicines. Remedicalization is an ongoing process, and how cannabis is treated is relevant to other psychoactive drugs with potential medical utility, such as LSD or psilocybin. What impact the debate will have on the later stages of remedicalization remains to be seen. In the end this is about more than cannabis. In an era when we are facing significant global threats from issues such as climate change, disruptions to food supply, and pandemics such as Covid-19, how we negotiate the science–policy interchange has never been more important.

Notes

INTRODUCTION

1 Potter and Weinstock, *High Time*.
2 WHO, Expert Committee on Drug Dependence, *Thirty-Ninth Report*.
3 INCB, *Report of the INCB for 2019*.
4 Seddon and Floodgate, *Regulating Cannabis*.
5 Blech, *Inventing Diseases and Pushing Pills*; Narrain and Chandran, *Nothing to Fix*; Zarhin, 'The Trajectory of "Medical Cannabis" in Israel'; Zarhin et al., '"Medical Cannabis" as a Contested Medicine'.
6 Merlin, *Man and Marijuana*.
7 Abel, *Marihuana: The First Twelve Thousand Years*.
8 Brunner, 'Marijuana in Ancient Greece and Rome?', 344–55.
9 Lewis, 'Historical Perspective', 241–5; Kalant, 'Report of the Indian Hemp Drugs Commission', 77–96.
10 Lewis, 'Historical Perspective', 241–5.
11 Solomon, *The Marijuana Papers*.
12 Booth, *Cannabis*; Matthews, *Cannabis Culture*.
13 Star and Griesemer, 'Institutional Ecology', 387–420.
14 Epstein, *Impure Science*.
15 Berridge, 'Changing Places', 11–34.
16 Berridge, *Marketing Health*, 138.
17 Berridge, 'Altered States', 656.
18 Sherratt, 'Peculiar Substances', 1–10.
19 Goode, 'Marijuana and the Politics of Reality', 83–94.
20 Ungerleider and Andrysiak, 'Bias and the Cannabis Researcher', S153–8.
21 Taylor and Berridge, 'Medicinal Plants for the Control and Treatment for Infectious Tropical Disease', 707–14.
22 Arber, *Herbals*.
23 Pickstone, 'Medical Botany', 94–5.
24 Schultes and von Reis, *Ethnobotany*.
25 Honigsbaum, *The Fever Trail*.

26 Dobson, 'Bittersweet Solutions'.

27 Powers, 'Drug Resistant Malaria', 262–87.

28 Goodman and Walsh, *The Story of Taxol.*

29 Healy, *The Creation of Psychopharmacology*; Tansey, Christie, and Reynolds, 'Drugs in Psychiatric Practice'.

30 Russo, *Cannabis: From Pariah to Prescription*, 2.

31 Kalant, 'Ludlow on Cannabis', 309–22; Glatt, 'Historical Note', 99–108; Hindmarch, 'A Social History', 252–7.

32 Berridge, *Opium and the People*, 209–15.

33 The pharmacopoeia were important because, prior to the 1968 Medicines Control Act, they provided the only control of medicines (other than those regarded as dangerous), setting quality standards for the preparation of drugs. The first *British Pharmacopoeia* was published in 1864. In 1907 it was supplemented by the *British Pharmaceutical Codex*, which supplied information on and provided standards for drugs and other pharmaceutical substances not included in the pharmacopoeia.

34 Mechoulam and Hanus, 'A Historical Overview of Chemical Research on Cannabinoids', 1–13.

35 Berridge, *Opium and the People*, 209–15.

36 Russo, 'History of Cannabis as a Medicine', 6.

37 Kalant, 'Report of the Indian Hemp Drugs Commission, 1893–94', 77–96.

38 Basu, 'Cannabis and Madness', 131–8.

39 Mills, *Madness, Cannabis and Colonialism.*

40 Guba, *Taming Cannabis.*

41 Edwards and Strang, 'Britain's Drug Crisis', *Independent*, 3 March 1994, https://bit.ly/3vZcZbt.

42 Musto, 'The 1937 Marijuana Tax Act', 101–8.

43 Saper, 'The Making of Policy', 183–93.

44 Mills, *Cannabis Britannica.*

45 WHO, Expert Committee on Drugs Liable to Produce Addiction. *Third Report*, 11.

46 Mills, *Cannabis Nation*, 87.

47 Brunn, *The Gentlemen's Club.*

48 Bewley-Taylor, *The United States and International Drug Control*; McAllister, *Drug Diplomacy.*

49 Abel, *Marihuana.*

50 Barker and Peters, *The Politics of Expert Advice.*

51 MacLeod, *Public Science and Public Policy.*

52 Berridge, *Marketing Health*, 133.

53 Bulmer, 'The Royal Commission and Departmental Committee', 37–49.

54 Lorway, AIDS *Activism, Science and Community*; Klawiter, *The Biopolitics of Breast Cancer*; Vicari and Cappai, 'Health Activism and the Logic of Connective Action'.

55 Mold, *Making the Patient-Consumer*.

56 Bone and Walden, 'New Trends in Illicit Cannabis Cultivation'; Klein and Potter, 'The Three Betrayals of the Medical Cannabis Growing Activist'.

57 Randall, 'Glaucoma', 99.

58 Dufton, *Grass Routes*.

59 Bock, *Waiting to Inhale*.

60 Newhart and Dolphin, *The Medicalization of Marijuana*.

61 Weatherall, *In Search of a Cure*.

62 Slinn, 'Research and Development in the UK Pharmaceutical Industry'.

63 Quirke, 'Collaboration in the Pharmaceutical Industry'.

64 Slinn, 'The Development of the Pharmaceutical Industry'.

65 Herzberg, *White Market Drugs*.

66 Mikuriya, 'Marijuana in Medicine', 34–40.

67 Russo, 'History of Cannabis as a Medicine'.

68 Casto, 'Marijuana and the Assassins', 747–55.

69 Berridge, 'Queen Victoria's Cannabis Use', 213–15.

70 Anderson, *Making Medicines*.

71 Perks and Thomson, *The Oral History Reader*.

72 Crowther *et al.*, *The Medicalization of Cannabis*.

73 Florin, 'Scientific Uncertainty', 1269–83.

CHAPTER ONE

1 Bloomquist, *Marijuana*; Matthews, *Cannabis Culture*; Booth, *Cannabis*.

2 CND, *The Question of Cannabis*.

3 Mechoulam and Hanus, 'A Historical Overview of Chemical Research', 1–13.

4 Raphael Mechoulam, interview by Suzanne Taylor.

5 Mechoulam and Gaoni, 'A Total Synthesis of dl-Delta-1-Tetrahydrocannabinol', 3273–5.

6 Stereochemistry: a sub-discipline of chemistry that involves the study of the relative spatial arrangement of atoms within molecules.

7   Roger Pertwee, interview by Suzanne Taylor.

8   Russo, *Cannabis: From Pariah to Prescription*, 2.

9   Organe, Paton, and Zamis, 'Preliminary Trials of
     Bistrimethylammonium Decane', 21–3.

10   Paton, 'Drug Dependence: A Socio-Pharmacological Assessment',
     200–12.

11   Healy, *The Creation of Psychopharmacy*; WHO, Expert Committee on
     Drugs Liable to Produce Addiction, *Report on the Second Session*, 273;
     Berridge, *Marketing Health*, 259.

12   Bewley-Taylor, 'The Drugs Problem of the 1960s', 43.

13   The model of dependence would receive wider support in the 1980s
     when a broader conception of dependence was adopted. See Hall,
     Cannabis Use and Dependence, 71.

14   Paton, 'Drug Dependence: A Socio-Pharmacological Assessment',
     200–12.

15   Edward Gill, quoted in Crowther *et al.*, *The Medicalization of Cannabis*.

16   Guy, Whittle, and Robson, *The Medicinal Uses of Cannabis and
     Cannabinoids*, 390.

17   McAllister, *Drug Diplomacy in the Twentieth Century*, 5.

18   WHO, Expert Committee on Drugs Liable to Produce Addiction,
     Third Report.

19   UNODC, *The Cannabis Problem: A Note on the Problem and the
     History of International Action* (Vienna: UNODC, 1962), available at
     https://www.unodc.org/unodc/en/data-and-analysis/bulletin/
     bulletin_1962-01-01_4_page005.html.

20   Whittle and Guy, 'Development of Cannabis-Based Medicine', 436.

21   Krejci, 'Hemp (*Cannabis sativa*): Antibiotic Drugs; II', 155–66;
     Kabelik, 'Hemp (*Cannabis sativa*): Antibiotic Drugs; I', 439–43; Krejci,
     'Antibacterial Action of Cannabis Indica', 500.

22   Economic and Social Council, *The Question of Cannabis*.

23   WHO, Expert Committee on Drugs Liable to Produce Addiction,
     Third Report.

24   UNODC, *The Cannabis Problem*.

25   Room *et al.*, *Cannabis Policy*, 76.

26   Advisory Committee on Drug Dependence, Hallucinogens Sub-
     committee, *Cannabis*.

27   Ibid., 'A Comparison of Cannabis with Other Drugs', point 66.

28   Witton, Mars, and DrugScope, *Cannabis and the Gateway Hypothesis*.

29   Advisory Committee on Drug Dependence, Hallucinogens
     Sub-committee, *Cannabis*.

30   Ibid., 'General Conclusion and Recommendations', point 99.

31   Ibid., points 98–9.

32   Ibid., points 72–3.

33   House of Lords debates, 23 January 1969, vol. 298, col. 1040.

34   Ibid.

35   Strang and Gossop, *Heroin Addiction and the British System*, 47.

36   Berridge, *Marketing Health*, 266.

37   Medical Research Council papers, meeting of the Chairmen and Secretaries of the Council, Working Parties on Drugs Dependence, 27 June 1969, FD 7/1581, The National Archives (TNA).

38   Medical Research Council papers, minutes of the MRC Conference into Research into Drug Dependence (held 15 December 1967), 17 January 1968, FD 7/875, TNA.

39   Medical Research Council papers, MRC Working Party on Biochemical Aspects of Drug Dependence: minutes of 1st meeting, 29 April 1968, FD 7/1580, TNA.

40   Sir William Paton Collection, Misuse of Drugs: Outline of Proposed Legislation, PP/WDP/F/4/1, Wellcome Library.

41   Sir William Paton Collection, letter from J. Faulkner, MRC, to W.D.M. Paton, 8 October 1969, PP/WDP/F/4/1, Wellcome Library.

42   Sir William Paton Collection, letter from J. Faulkner, MRC, to D.G. Turner, Home Office, 25 November 1969, PP/WDP/F/4/1, Wellcome Library.

43   Sir William Paton Collection, letter from W.D.M. Paton to J. Faulkner, MRC, 7 November 1969, PP/WDP/F/4, Wellcome Library; see also Sir William Paton Collection, Comments on Proposed Legislation on Misuse of Drugs, background notes, PP/WDP/F/4, Wellcome Library.

44   Sir William Paton Collection, letter from W.D.M. Paton to J. Faulkner, MRC, 7 November 1969, PP/WDP/F/4, Wellcome Library.

45   Ibid.

46   Medical Research Council papers, MRC Working Party on Biochemical Aspects of Drug Dependence: minutes of 1st meeting, 29 April 1968, FD 7/1580, TNA.

47   Medical Research Council papers, minutes of the MRC Working Party on Biological and Pharmacological Aspects of Drug Dependence, 7 July 1969, FD 7/875, TNA.

48   Sir William Paton Collection, details of the Working Party on the Epidemiology of Drug Dependence, September 1969, PP/WDP/F/4/1, Wellcome Library.

49 Sir William Paton Collection, draft report of the Working Party on the Epidemiology of Drug Dependence, PP/WDP/F/4/1 Wellcome Library.

50 Sir William Paton Collection, meeting of the Chairmen and Secretaries of the Councils, Working Parties on Drug Dependence, 7 July 1969, PP/WDP/F/4/1, Wellcome Library.

51 Sir William Paton Collection, report of the Working Parties on Drug Dependence, office note, 17 June 1970, PP/WDP/F/4/4, Wellcome Library.

52 Sir William Paton Collection, Working Party on the Biological Aspects of Drug Dependence, MRC circulation, minutes of the first meeting, 6 July 1971, PP/WDP/F/4/7, Wellcome Library.

53 Sir William Paton Collection, letter from K. Levy, MRC, to W.D.M. Paton, 8 February 1971, PP/WDP/F/4/4, Wellcome Library.

54 Berridge, *Marketing Health*, 266.

55 Ibid., 3.

56 Paton, 'The Contribution of Classical Pharmacological Methods',

57 Edward Gill and Geoffrey Guy, quoted in Crowther *et al.*, *The Medicalization of Cannabis*.

58 Carson, *Silent Spring*.

59 Anderson, ed., *Making Medicines*.

60 Edward Gill, quoted in Crowther *et al.*, *The Medicalization of Cannabis*.

61 Medical Research Council papers, MRC Annual Report 1970/1, FD 7/881, TNA.

62 Sir William Paton Collection, letter from F. Ames to W.D.M. Paton, 21 September 1971; letter from R. Mechoulam to W.D.M. Paton, 27 April 1969; PP/WDP/F/1/1, Wellcome Library.

63 Sir William Paton Collection, letter from W.D.M. Paton to Mechoulam, 21 May 1969, PP/WDP/F/3, Wellcome Library.

64 Sir William Paton Collection, letter from K.L. Allford, Home Office, to Paton, 15 May 1969, PP/WDP/F/3, Wellcome Library.

65 Sir William Paton Collection, letter from R. Mechoulam to W.D.M. Paton, 27 April, 1969, PP/WDP/F/3, Wellcome Library.

66 McAllister, *Drug Diplomacy*, 201.

67 Medical Research Council papers, letter from Wrighton to W.D.M. Paton, 7 September 1971, FD 7/881, TNA.

68 Medical Research Council papers, Wrighton, notes, 15 October 1971, FD 7/881, TNA.

69 Medical Research Council papers, letter from R.J. Wrighton, MRC, to Dr H.O.J. Collier, Miles Laboratories Ltd, 25 May 1971, FD 7/881, TNA.

70 Medical Research Council papers, letter from W.D.M. Paton to Wrighton, MRC, 9 September 1971, FD 7/881, TNA.

71 Ibid.

72 Medical Research Council papers, letter from W.D.M. Paton to J. Faulkner, MRC, 4 November 1971, FD 7/881, TNA.

73 Medical Research Council papers, letter from W.D.M. Paton to J. Faulkner, MRC, 15 November 1971, FD 7/881, TNA.

74 Ibid.

75 Medical Research Council papers, letter from J. Isbister, NIMH, to Gray, MRC, 28 February 1972, FD 7/881, TNA.

76 Medical Research Council papers, letter from L.J. Hale to Dr King, 14 March 1972, FD 7/881, TNA.

77 Medical Research Council papers, letter from E.W. Gill to Simpson, 12 October 1973, FD 7/882, TNA.

78 Roger Pertwee, quoted in Crowther et al., The Medicalization of Cannabis.

79 Kosviner, Hawks, and Webb, 'Cannabis Use Amongst British University Students', 35–60.

80 Paton, 'The Contribution of Classical Pharmacological Methods',

81 Pertwee, 'Cannabinoid Pharmacology'.

82 Ibid.

83 Gill, Paton, and Pertwee, 'Preliminary Experiments on the Chemistry and Pharmacology of Cannabis', 134–6.

84 Loewe, 'The Active Principles of Cannabis', 175–93.

85 Pertwee, interview.

86 Pertwee, 'Cannabinoid Pharmacology', S163–71.

87 Pertwee 'The Ring Test', 753–63.

88 Berridge, Marketing Health, 268.

89 Edward Gill, quoted in Crowther et al., The Medicalization of Cannabis.

90 Gill, Paton, and Pertwee, 'Preliminary Experiments on the Chemistry and Pharmacology of Cannabis', 134–6; Paton, 'Additional Remarks on the Chronic Toxicity of Cannabis', 617–18; Paton and Pertwee, 'The Actions of Cannabis in Man', 287–333.

91 Teratogenicity: the ability to disturb the growth and development of an embryo or foetus.

92 Paton, 'Drug Dependence: Pharmacological and Physiological Aspects', 247–54.

93 Ibid.

94 Paton, 'Achievements Resulting From Animal Research', 16–25.

95 Paton, Cannabis and Related Drugs, 105–24

96 Sir William Paton Collection, letter from W.D.M. Paton to
    Dr Weatherall, Senior Medical Statistician, Office of Population
    Censuses and Surveys, 21 August 1981, PP/WDP/F/3, Wellcome
    Library.
97 Paton, 'Drug Dependence: A Socio-Pharmacological Assessment',
    200–12.
98 Paton, *Cannabis and Related Drugs*, 105–24.
99 Ibid.
100 Paton, 'Molecular Basis of Drug Toxicity', 1–6.
101 Pertwee, 'Cannabinoid Pharmacology', S163–71; Pertwee, interview.
102 Mechoulam, interview.
103 Paton, 'Drug Dependence: A Socio-Pharmacological Assessment',
    200.
104 Healy, *The Creation of Psychopharmacy*, 362.
105 Tylden and Paton, 'Clinical Aspects of Cannabis Action', 362.
106 Sir William Paton Collection, letter from G. Nahas to W.D.M. Paton,
    2 April 1971, PP/WDP/F/1/14, Wellcome Library.
107 Sir William Paton Collection, letter from G. Nahas to W.D.M. Paton,
    12 February 1973, PP/WDP/F/1/14, Wellcome Library.
108 Nahas, *Keep off the Grass*.
109 Sir William Paton Collection, letter from W.D.M. Paton to
    D. Laurence, 9 April 1973, PP/WDP/F/1/14, Wellcome Library.
110 Sir William Paton Collection, letter from Springer Verlag to G. Nahas,
    19 August 1976, PP/WDP/F/1/14, Wellcome Library.
111 Sir William Paton Collection, letter from W.D.M Paton to
    R. Mechoulam, 14 June 1974, PP/WDP/F/3, Wellcome Library.
112 Edward Gill, quoted in Crowther *et al.*, *The Medicalization of Cannabis*.
113 Paton, 'Cell Pathological Effects of Cannabis', 340.
114 Sir William Paton Collection, letter from W.D.M. Paton to Ms Boyle,
    CRC Press Inc., 9 February 1983, PP/WDP/F/3, Wellcome Library.
115 Paton, 'Drug Dependence: A Socio-Pharmacological Assessment',
    200.
116 Sir William Paton Collection, letter from W.D.M. Paton to
    R. Mechoulam, 1 September 1981, PP/WDP/F/3, Wellcome Library.
117 Sir William Paton Collection, letter from W.D.M Paton to
    Ms Boyle, CRC Press Inc., 9 February 1983, PP/WDP/F/3,
    Wellcome Library.
118 Paton, 'The Contribution of Classical Pharmacological Methods'.
119 Paton, 'Pharmacology'.

CHAPTER TWO

1　Graham, 'If Cannabis Were a New Drug', 417–37.
2　Mechoulam and Hanus, 'A Historical Overview of Chemical Research', 8.
3　Petersen, *Marihuana Research Findings*, 200.
4　Randall, 'Glaucoma: A Patient's View', 94–102.
5　Hepler and Frank, 'Marihuana Smoking and Intraocular Pressure', 1,392.
6　Hepler, Frank, and Petrus, 'Ocular Effects of Marihuana Smoking', 815–24.
7　Sir William Paton Collection, letter from R. Mechoulam to W.D.M. Paton, 19 December 1976, PP/WDP/F/3, Wellcome Library.
8　Ibid.
9　Sir William Paton Collection, letter from R. Mechoulam to W.D.M. Paton, 25 May 1978, PP/WDP/F/3, Wellcome Library.
10　Ibid.
11　US Department of Health and Human Services, *Investigation of Possible Medical Uses of Marijuana*, HHS Fact Sheet, 13 July 1999, archived version (from 24 February 1999) available from https://bit.ly/3HJVwIv.
12　Noyes *et al.*, 'Analgesic Effect of Delta-9-Tetrahydrocannabinol', 139–43; Noyes *et al.*, 'The Analgesic Properties of Delta-9-Tetrahydrocannabinol', 84–9; Raft *et al.*, 'Effects of Intravenous Tetrahydrocannabinol', 26–33.
13　Goodman and Walsh, *The Story of Taxol*.
14　Mead, 'International Control of Cannabis', 382.
15　Sallan, Zinberg, and Frei, 'Antiemetic Effect of Delta-9-THC', 795–7.
16　Chang *et al.*, 'Delta-9-Tetrahydrocannabinol as an Antiemetic', 819–24.
17　For a review of the trials see Iverson, *The Science of Marijuana*.
18　Sir William Paton Collection, letter from R. Mechoulam to W.D.M. Paton, 25 May 1978, PP/WDP/F/3, Wellcome Library.
19　Graham, 'The Effect of Delta1-Tetrahydrocannabinol', 465–6.
20　Spriggs, 'J.D.P. Graham', 3–4.
21　Graham, 'The 2-Halogenoalkylamines', 132–71; Graham and James, 'The Pharmacology of a Series', 489–504; Graham and al Katib, 'The Action of Trypsin', 1–14.
22　Graham and Li, 'Cardiovascular and Respiratory Effects', 1–10.

23   Graham, 'Cannabis and the Cardiovascular System', 857.

24   Autonomic pharmacology: the study of drugs related to the autonomic nervous system. Broncholidation refers to a drug widening the air passages of the lungs and eases breathing by relaxing bronchial smooth muscle, and bronchodilators are the means of administering the drug.

25   An analogue is a drug whose structure is related to that of another drug but whose chemical and biological properties may be quite different.

26   Barnes, 'Drugs for Asthma', S297–303.

27   Clark, 'Medical Aerosol Inhalers', 374–91.

28   Hartley, Nogrady, and Seaton, 'Bronchodilator Effect of Delta1-Tetrahydrocannabinol', 523–5

29   Williams, Hartley, and Graham, 'Bronchodilator Effect of Delta1-Tetrahydrocannabinol Administered by Aerosol', 720–3.

30   Nahas, *Biomedical Aspects of Cannabis Usage*.

31   Ibid.

32   Graham, 'The Bronchodilator Action of Cannabinoids',

33   Davies, Weatherstone, and Graham, 'A Pilot Study of Orally Administered Delta Nine Trans THC', 301–6.

34   Ibid.

35   Ibid.

36   Graham, 'If Cannabis Were a New Drug', 417–37.

37   Graham, *Cannabis Now*, 59.

38   Woodcock, 'Cannabis Now', 248.

39   Graham, *Cannabis Now*.

40   Ibid., 35.

41   Berridge, *Marketing Health*, 16–17.

42   Graham, *Cannabis Now*, 61.

43   Home Office papers, minutes of the Working Group on Cannabis, 18th meeting, 3 February 1977, HO 319/178, TNA.

44   Home Office papers, minutes of the Working Group, 13th meeting, 9 July 1975, HO 319/172, TNA.

45   Home Office papers, minutes of the Working Group, 5th meeting, 19 September 1973, HO 319/166, TNA.

46   Ibid.

47   *The Lancet*, 'The Therapeutic Possibilities in Cannabinoids', 667–9.

48   Nahas, *Biomedical Aspects of Cannabis Usage*.

49   Ibid.

50   Cohen, 'Therapeutic Aspects', 194.

51 Ibid.

52 Sir William Paton Collection, letter from Ames to W.D.M. Paton, 23 April 1975, PP/WDP/F/1/1.F, Wellcome Library.

53 Cohen, 'Therapeutic Aspects', 194.

54 Ministry of Health papers, report of the Expert Group on the Effects of Cannabis Use, 1982, ACMD Working Group on Cannabis, MH 149/1946, TNA.

55 Rose, 'Cannabis: A Medical Question?', 703.

56 Rose, 'Cannabis and the Rule of Law', 138.

57 Ibid.

58 Ibid.

59 Ibid., 139.

60 Ibid., 138.

61 Anno, 'Cannabinoids for Nausea', 255–6.

62 DuQuesne, 'Cannabis and the Rule of Law', 581.

63 Healy, *The Creation of Psychopharmacology*, 163.

64 Ministry of Health papers, press cuttings, 1980–82, MH 149/1946, TNA.

65 Ministry of Health papers, 'Use of Cannabis by Cancer Patients', revised brief, from Sir Henry Eylloless, Chief Medical Officer, to Mr Knight, MH 149/1946, TNA.

66 *The Lancet* [Gerard Vaughan (Minister of Health)?], 'Government Policy on Cannabis', 574.

67 Letter from Rose to J.D.P. Graham, 16 February 1981, Graham's personal papers.

68 Sir William Paton Collection, letter from W.D.M. Paton to Dr Harwick, Home Office, 24 September 1981, PP/WDP/F/3, Wellcome Library.

69 Sir William Paton Collection, letter from Dr D. Black, Senior Medical Office, DHSS, to W.D.M. Paton, 19 October 1981, PP/WDP/F/3, Wellcome Library.

70 Iverson, *The Science of Marijuana*, 143.

71 Pertwee, interview.

72 Ibid.

73 Ibid.

74 Cohen, 'Therapeutic Aspects'.

75 Medical Research Council papers, Addiction Review Group Report, PP/WDP/F/4/13, Wellcome Library.

76 House of Commons debates, Drug Misuse, 8 December 1989, vol. 163, col. 594.

77 Pertwee, interview.
78 Sir William Paton Collection, letter from W.D.M. Paton to Boyle, 9 February 1983, PP/WDP/F/3, Wellcome Library.
79 Pertwee, interview.
80 Sir William Paton Collection, letter from R. Mechoulam to W.D.M. Paton, 27 April, 1969, pp/wdp/f3, Wellcome Library
81 Hughes *et al.*, 'Identification of Two Related Pentapeptides', 577–80.
82 The vas deferens is a coiled duct that conveys sperms from the epididymis to the ejaculatory duct and the urethra.

CHAPTER THREE

1   Berridge, *Marketing Health.*
2   Barker and Peters, *The Politics of Expert Advice.*
3   MacLeod, *Public Science and Public Policy.*
4   Hamlin, 'Expert Witnessing'.
5   Berridge, *Marketing Health.*
6   Ibid., 153.
7   Bulmer, 'The Royal Commission and Departmental Committee'.
8   Home Office papers, ACMD, minutes of the 1st meeting of the Working Group on Cannabis, 1 December 1972, HO 319/162, TNA.
9   Spriggs, 'J.D.P. Graham', 3–4.
10 Griffith Edwards, quoted in Crowther *et al.*, *The Medicalization of Cannabis.*
11 Home Office papers, G. Edwards, 'Cannabis and the Criteria for Legalisation of a Currently Prohibited Recreational Drug: Groundwork for a Debate', 1973, HO 319/166, TNA.
12 Home Office papers, ACMD, minutes of the 5th meeting of the Working Group on Cannabis, 19 September 1973, HO 319/175, TNA.
13 Sherratt, 'Peculiar Substances', 1–10.
14 Home Office papers, ACMD, minutes of the 15th meeting of the Working Group on Cannabis, 22 October 1975, HO 319/175, TNA.
15 Home Office papers, ACMD, Biochemical and Pharmacological Studies, minutes of the 3rd meeting of the Working Group on Cannabis, 23 May 1973, HO 319/166, TNA.
16 Home Office papers, ACMD, minutes of the 5th meeting of the Working Group on Cannabis, 19 September 1973, HO 319/175, TNA.
17 Ibid.
18 Home Office papers, ACMD, Attachment to First Interim Report of the Working Group on Cannabis, Bloomfield, December 1973, HO 319/166, TNA.

19 Jasanoff, *The Fifth Branch.*

20 Ibid.

21 Ibid.

22 Hilgartner, *Science on Stage.*

23 Florin, *How Does Science Influence Policy?*

24 Home Office papers, letter from Mr T.D. McCaffrey, Public Relations Branch, to Mr Stotesbury, 14 January 1974, HO 319/167, TNA.

25 Home Office papers, note by Mr Stotesbury, Probation and After-Care Department, ACMD Working Group on Cannabis First Interim Report, 3 January 1974, HO 319/167, TNA.

26 Home Office papers, ACMD, minutes of the 9th meeting of the Working Group on Cannabis, 27 March 1974, HO 319/144, TNA.

27 Home Office papers, ACMD, minutes of the 11th meeting of the Working Group on Cannabis, 27 September 1974, HO 319/170, TNA.

28 Home Office papers, minutes of the 13th meeting of the Working Group on Cannabis, paper presented to the working group by J.D.P. Graham, 'Therapeutic Possibilities in Cannabinoids', 9 July 1975, HO 319/172, TNA.

29 Home Office papers, ACMD, minutes of the 8th meeting of the Working Group on Cannabis, item four, paper from the Home Office on the 'Effects of Statutory Controls on the Use of Cannabis', 8 February 1974, HO 319/168, TNA.

30 Home Office papers, minutes of the 5th meeting of the Working Group on Cannabis, 22 October 1975, HO 319/175, TNA.

31 Ministry of Health papers, Reservation and Alternative Conclusions to the Second Interim Report, MH 149/1946, TNA.

32 Ibid.

33 Home Office papers, note from Mr D.I. de Deney, Home Office, 15 January 1976, HO 319/174, TNA.

34 Home Office papers, press cuttings, drug report, 'Back into the Melting Pot', *New Scientist*, 2 December 1976, HO 319/174, TNA.

35 Home Office, ACMD, minutes of the 17th meeting of the Working Group on Cannabis, 26 November 1976, HO 319/177, TNA.

36 Ibid.

37 Home Office papers, letter from de Deney to Mr Glanville, 6 May 1976, HO 319/174, TNA.

38 Home Office papers, ACMD, Response to Second Interim Report, March 1976, HO 319/174 TNA.

39 Ministry of Health papers, ACMD, Expert Group on the Effects of Cannabis, report, 1982, MH 149/1946, TNA.

40 Ibid.

41 Ibid.

42 Home Office papers, minutes of the 18th meeting of the Working Group on Cannabis, paper presented by J.D.P. Graham, 'The Long Term Effects of Cannabis on the Health of Man', 3 February 2977, HO 319/178, TNA.

43 Home Office papers, ACMD, minutes of the 2nd meeting of the ACMD Technical Sub-committee, September 1974, HO 319/199, TNA.

44 Ministry of Health papers, ACMD, meeting of the Technical Sub-committee, 1977, MH149/1945, TNA.

45 Home Office papers, letter from G. Edwards to J. Bloomfield, 14 March 1977, HO 319/180, TNA.

46 Home Office papers, ACMD, minutes of the 19th meeting of the Working Group on Cannabis, 28 February 1977, HO 319/179, TNA.

47 Ibid. Home Office papers, letter from J. Bloomfield to G. Edwards, 16 March 1977, HO 319/180, TNA.

48 Home Office papers, ACMD, minutes of the 19th meeting of the Working Group on Cannabis, 28 February 1977, HO 319/179, TNA.

49 Home Office papers, ACMD, minutes of the 12th meeting of the Technical Sub-committee, 1978, HO 319/209. TNA.

50 Ministry of Health papers, ACMD, meeting of the Technical Sub-committee, 1977, MH149/1945, TNA.

51 Ministry of Health papers, ACMD, report of the Expert Group on the Effects of Cannabis Use, September 1981, MH 149/1946, TNA.

52 Ministry of Health papers, ACMD, government response, 1981, TNA.

53 Ministry of Health papers, release, 'Trash Rehashed: A Reply to the ACMD', MH 149/1946, TNA.

54 Ministry of Health papers, ACMD, report of the Expert Group on the Effects of Cannabis Use, September 1981, MH 149/1946, TNA.

55 Ibid.

56 Ibid.

57 Ministry of Health papers, Chief Medical Office, note [17 July 1980?], MH 149/1946, TNA.

58 ARF/WHO, *Cannabis and Health Hazards.*

59 Ministry of Health papers, ACMD, minutes of meeting of the Expert Group on the Effects of Cannabis Use, 28 August 1980, MH 149/1946, TNA.

60 Ibid.

61 Ministry of Health papers, ACMD, draft press note, 1982, MH 149/1946, TNA.

62 Ministry of Health papers, ACMD, minutes of meeting of the Expert Group on the Effects of Cannabis Use, 28 August 1980, MH 149/1946, TNA.

63 Ibid.

64 Ministry of Health papers, ACMD, letter from D.J. Hardwick to members of the ACMD, 16 March 1982, MH 149/1946, TNA.

65 Ministry of Health papers, ACMD, draft press note, 1982, MH 149/1946, TNA.

66 Ministry of Health papers, ACMD, 'Therapeutic Use of Cannabis', note of a meeting held on 15 February 1982, MH 149/1946, TNA.

67 Jasanoff, *Fifth Branch*.

CHAPTER FOUR

1 Slinn, 'Research and Development in the UK', 186; Hill-Curth, *From Physick to Pharmacology*.

2 Slinn, 'The Development of the Pharmaceutical Industry', 155–76.

3 Quirke, 'From Alkaloids to Gene Therapy', 177–201.

4 Goodman and Walsh, *The Story of Taxol*, 144.

5 Mechoulam, interview.

6 K. Coe, reported by Iverson, 'Notes on Conference "Marihuana and Medicine" at New York University Medical Center, New York, 20–1 March 1998', in House of Lords Select Committee on Science and Technology, *Cannabis: The Scientific and Medical Evidence*, appendix 3.

7 Slinn, 'Research and Development', 170.

8 Mathre, 'Cannabis Series: The Whole Story; Part 4'; Mathre, 'Cannabis Series. The Whole Story; Part 5'; Iverson, *The Science of Marijuana*, 143.

9 BMA, *Therapeutic Uses of Cannabis*, 22.

10 FDA, 'Potential Merits of Cannabinoids for Medical Uses', FDA website, archived version (from 5 March 2010) available from https://bit.ly/3Nqx7Jf.

11 An isomer is a compound with the same molecular formula but a different structural formula. For instance, the compound contains the same number of atoms of the same elements but these are arranged in a different structure, thereby providing different properties.

12 McAllister, *Drug Diplomacy*, 230

13 Iverson, *The Science of Marijuana*, 144.

14 Ibid.

15 Since 2000 these drugs have experienced something of a revival.
    Nabilone was bought by Valeant Pharmaceuticals from Eli Lilly and
    approved by the FDA in 2006, and in 2007 Valeant Pharmaceuticals
    acquired the rights from Cambridge Laboratories to market Nabilone
    in the United Kingdom.

16 WHO, Expert Committee on Drugs Liable to Produce Addiction,
    Twenty-Sixth Report.

17 Quirke, 'From Alkaloids to Gene Therapy', 197.

18 Slinn, 'The Development of the Pharmaceutical Industry', 93.

19 Pertwee, interview.

20 Ibid.

21 Endogenous refers to substances that originate within an organism.
    In relation to cannabinoids, this essentially means substances that
    originate in the human body rather than the plant.

22 Hill, 'G-Protein-Coupled Receptors', S27–37.

23 Pertwee, interview. G-protein-coupled receptors are cell surface
    receptors that bind to G proteins and are involved in chemical
    signalling between nerve cells.

24 Hill, 'G-Protein-Coupled Receptors', S27–37.

25 Pertwee, 'Cannabinoid Pharmacology', S169.

26 Pertwee, interview.

27 In biochemistry, a receptor is a protein molecule, embedded in
    either the plasma membrane or the cytoplasm of a cell, to which one
    or more specific kinds of signaling molecules may attach. A molecule
    that binds (attaches) to a receptor is called a ligand. Each kind of
    receptor can bind only certain ligand shapes. Each cell typically has
    many receptors, of many different kinds.

28 Devane *et al.*, 'Determination and Characterization', 605–13.

29 Pertwee, interview.

30 Ibid.

31 Rang, 'The Receptor Concept', S9–16.

32 Pertwee, interview.

33 Ibid.

34 An agonist is a type of ligand that binds and alters the activity of a
    receptor.

35 Mechoulam, interview.

36 Ibid.

37 Rang, 'The Receptor Concept', S9–16.

38 Pertwee, interview.

39 Mechoulam, interview.

40 Devane *et al.*, 'Isolation and Structure', 1,946–9.

41 Pertwee, interview.

42 Ibid.

43 Ibid.

44 Vincenzo di Marzio, quoted in Crowther *et al.*, *The Medicalization of Cannabis.*

45 Mechoulam, interview.

46 Lesley Iverson, interview by Suzanne Taylor.

47 An allosteric site is a site on an enzyme molecule that binds with a non-substrate molecule, inducing a conformational change that results in an alteration of the affinity of the enzyme for its substrate.

48 Pertwee, interview.

49 Iverson, interview

50 Ibid.

51 Pertwee, interview.

52 Vincenzo di Marzio, quoted in Crowther *et al.*, *The Medicalization of Cannabis*, 44.

53 WHO, Expert Committee on Drug Dependence, *Twenty-Seventh Report*, 11.

54 Ibid., 12.

55 Ibid.

56 Room *et al.*, *Cannabis Policy*, 11.

57 Iverson, *The Science of Marijuana*, 135.

58 Robson and Guy, 'Clinical Studies of Cannabis-Based Medicines', 230.

59 Taylor and Berridge, 'Medicinal Plants for the Control', 707–14.

60 Ibid.

61 Mead, 'International Control of Cannabis', 407.

62 Taylor and Berridge, 'Medicinal Plants for the Control and Treatment of Infectious Tropical Disease', 707–14.

63 WHO, *Traditional Medicine and Modern Health Care*, 4.

64 IUCN, WHO, and WWF, *Guidelines on the Conservation.*

65 WHO, *Traditional Medicine and Modern*, 4; WHO, *Progress Report by the Director-General*, 22 March 1991 (Geneva: WHO).

66 Goodman and Walsh, *The Story of Taxol*, 232.

67 Guy, 'Introduction', xxii.

68 Slinn, 'The Development of the Pharmaceutical Industry', 170.

69 Quirke, 'From Alkaloids to Gene Therapy', 197.

70 Ibid.

71 Dunlop, 'Legislation on Medicines', 760–2; Tansey *et al.*, *The Committee on Safety of Drugs*, 103–35.

72 Geoffrey Guy, quoted in Crowther *et al.*, *The Medicalization of Cannabis*, 30.

73 Kirby, 'Medicinal Plants and the Control of Protozoal Disease', 605–9. Taylor and Berridge, 'Medicinal Plants for the Control and Treatment of Infectious Tropical Disease', 707–14; Chawira *et al.*, 'The Effect of Combination', 554–58; London School of Hygiene and Tropical Medicine, *Annual Report*, 59.

74 Oudshoorn, 'United We Stand', 345.

75 Lowy and Gaudilliere, *The Invisible Industrialist*, 21.

76 Pertwee, interview.

77 Geoffrey Guy, quoted in Crowther *et al.*, *The Medicalization of Cannabis*, 36.

78 Phillip Robson, interview by Suzanne Taylor.

79 Geoffrey Guy, quoted in Crowther *et al.*, *The Medicalization of Cannabis*, 31.

80 Robson, interview.

81 Geoffrey Guy, quoted in Crowther *et al.*, *The Medicalization of Cannabis*, 35.

82 House of Lords Select Committee on Science and Technology, *Cannabis: The Scientific and Medical Evidence*.

83 Robson, interview.

84 Home Affairs Select Committee, Minutes of Evidence Taken before the Home Affairs Committee, Session 2001-02, on the Work of the Home Office, HC 302, Q. 5.

85 Griffith Edwards, quoted in Crowther *et al.*, *The Medicalization of Cannabis*, 29.

86 Geoffrey Guy, quoted in Crowther *et al.*, *The Medicalization of Cannabis*, 39.

87 Ibid.

88 Ibid.

89 David Potter, interview by Suzanne Taylor.

90 Lowy and Gaudilliere, *The Invisible Industrialists*, 6.

91 Goodman and Walsh, *The Story of Taxol*, 117.

92 Potter, interview.

93 Potter, 'Growth and Morphology of Medicinal Cannabis', 29.

94 Russo, *Cannabis: From Pariah to Prescription*, 7.

95 Shiva, *Biopiracy*.

96 Booth, *Cannabis*, 299.

97 Potter, interview.

98 Ibid.

99 Guy, Whittle, and Robson, *The Medicinal Uses of Cannabis*, 274.

100 Notcutt, quoted in Crowther *et al.*, *The Medicalization of Cannabis*, 57.

CHAPTER FIVE

1   Berridge. *Marketing Health.*

2   Abrams, 'Cannabis Law Reform in Britain', 69–79.

3   SOMA, 'The Law Against Marijuana Is Immoral in Principle and Unworkable in Practice'.

4   Abrams, 'The Wootton Report'. Advisory Committee on Drug Dependence, Hallucinogen Sub-committee, *Cannabis.*

5   Wood, *Patient Power?*

6   Dufton, *Grass Routes.*

7   Randall, 'Glaucoma: A Patient's View', 94–102.

8   Home Office papers, minutes of the Working Group on Cannabis, 18th meeting, 3 February 1977, HO 319/178. TNA.

9   Werner, 'Medical Marijuana and the AIDS Crisis', 32.

10 Booth, *Cannabis.*

11 Clare Hodges (Clare Brice), interview by Suzanne Taylor.

12 Mead, 'International Control of Cannabis', 44–64.

13 House of Lords Select Committee on Science and Technology, *Cannabis: The Scientific and Medical Evidence; Evidence*, 90.

14 John Zajicek, interview by Suzanne Taylor.

15 Hodges, interview.

16 Wood, *Patient Power?*

17 Hodges, interview.

18 Mathre, *Cannabis in Medical Practice.*

19 Hodges, interview.

20 Wood, *Patient Power?*

21 Hodges, interview.

22 William Notcutt, interview by Suzanne Taylor.

23 Hodges, interview.

24 Ibid.

25 Ibid.

26 Lorna Layward, interview by Suzanne Taylor.

27 Boycott, 'Why We Believe It Is Time to Decriminalise Cannabis', *Independent*, 28 September 1997, https://bit.ly/3M3T2Wu.

28 Wood, *Patient Power?*
29 Nicolson and Lowis, 'The Early History of the Multiple Sclerosis Society of Great Britain and Northern Ireland: A Socio-Historical Study of Lay/Practitioner Interaction in the Context of a Medical Charity'.
30 Layward, interview.
31 Ibid.
32 Ibid.
33 Wood, *Patient Power?*
34 Mechoulam and Hanus, 'A Historical Overview of Chemical Research on Cannabinoids', 1–13.
35 Layward, interview.
36 David Baker, quoted in Crowther *et al.*, *The Medicalization of Cannabis*, 51–3.
37 Layward, interview.
38 Baker *et al.*, 'Cannabinoids Control Spasticity and Tremor in a Multiple Sclerosis Model', 84–7.
39 BBC, 'Cannabis "Helps MS Sufferers"', BBC, 2 March 2000, https://bbc.in/37wMSPP.
40 Baker, quoted in Crowther *et al.*, *The Medicalization of Cannabis*, 53.
41 House of Lords Select Committee on Science and Technology, *Cannabis: The Scientific and Medical Evidence*, 90.
42 Ibid., 9.
43 Ibid., 10.
44 Layward, interview.
45 RPS and MS Society, 'Therapeutic Applications of Cannabinoids', 130–1.
46 Layward, interview.
47 House of Lords Select Committee on Science and Technology, *Cannabis: The Scientific and Medical Evidence*, 40.
48 BMA, *Therapeutic Uses of Cannabis*.
49 Layward, interview.
50 Farmer, 'Court Clears MS Patient Who Used Cannabis Openly', *Independent*, 18 March 2000.
51 Hodges, interview.
52 Berridge, *Marketing Health*, 164.
53 Ibid.
54 House of Lords Select Committee on Science and Technology, *Cannabis: The Scientific and Medical Evidence*, 44–9.

55 All Party Parliamentary Group for MS, Meeting of the All Party Parliamentary Group for MS, 24 February 2004 (document removed from website by July 2019; a copy is in the author's personal archive).

56 House of Lords Select Committee on Science and Technology, *Cannabis: The Scientific and Medical Evidence*, 27–32, 84–100.

57 Ibid., 84–100.

58 Robson, interview.

59 Layward, interview.

60 House of Lords Select Committee on Science and Technology, *Cannabis: The Scientific and Medical Evidence*, 173–82.

61 Robson, interview.

62 House of Lords Select Committee on Science and Technology, *Cannabis: The Scientific and Medical Evidence*, 173–82.

63 Ibid., 30.

64 Ibid., 28.

65 Ibid., 30.

66 Hodges, interview.

CHAPTER SIX

1 Room *et al.*, *Cannabis Policy*.

2 House of Commons debates, 1 November 1994, vol. 248, col. 1064; House of Commons debates, Cannabis (Therapeutic Use), 12 July 1995, vol. 263, cols. 921–8.

3 House of Lords Select Committee on Science and Technology, *Cannabis: The Scientific and Medical Evidence; Evidence*, 49.

4 Ashton, *Cannabis: The Clinical and Pharmacological Aspects*; Robson, 'Therapeutic Aspects of Cannabis', 107–15.

5 Boycott, 'Why We Believe It Is Time to Decriminalise Cannabis', *Independent on Sunday*, 28 September 1997, https://bit.ly/3988ZN1.

6 Blackhurst and Routledge, 'Huge Majority Want Cannabis Legalised', *Independent on Sunday*, 12 October 1997, https://bit.ly/3N2nCjj; Ball, 'New Poll Reveals MPs in Favour of Change in Law on Drugs', *Independent on Sunday*, 2 November 1997.

7 Home Office, *Tackling Drugs to Build a Better Britain*.

8 WHO, *Cannabis*: Health Perspective and Research Agenda.

9 Ibid., 28.

10 Ibid.

11   Concar, 'High Anxieties'; BBC, 'Cannabis Safer than Alcohol and Tobacco', *BBC*, 19 February 1998, https://bbc.in/3sp8jcW.

12   WHO, *WHO Did Not Bow To Political Pressure in Publishing the Report on Cannabis*, press release, 19 February 1998, achived version (from 18 February 1999) available from https://bit.ly/3bj7JHY.

13   Trace, Klein, and Roberts, *Reclassification of Cannabis in the United Kingdom.*

14   BMA, *The Therapeutic Uses of Cannabis*, 2.

15   Ibid., 78.

16   BMA, 'An Outline History of the BMA', BMA website, http://www.bma. org.uk/about_bma/history/BMAOutlineHistory.jsp (accessed 10 July 2009; URL no longer active).

17   BMA, 'Science Board', BMA website, http://www.bma.org.uk/ representation/pro_committees/board_science/index.jsp (accessed 10 July 2009; URL no longer active).

18   BMA, *The Therapeutic Uses of Cannabis*, 1–2.

19   Sarah Mars, interview by Virginia Berridge and Suzanne Taylor.

20   BMA, *The Therapeutic Uses of Cannabis*, 2.

21   Ibid., 3.

22   BMA, *The Misuse of Drugs.*

23   Mars, interview.

24   Ibid.

25   Ibid.

26   BMA, *The Therapeutic Uses of Cannabis*, 77.

27   Ibid., 79.

28   Ibid.

29   Mars, interview.

30   Ibid.

31   BMA, *The Therapeutic Uses of Cannabis*, 78.

32   Mars, interview.

33   BMA, *BMA Report Calls for Change in Law and Development of New Cannabis-Based Medicines*, press release, 18 November 1997, available from https://bit.ly/39QnJAp (accessed 10 July 2009).

34   BBC, 'British Doctors Back Use of Cannabis', *BBC*, 19 November 1997, https://bbc.in/39Jv3gZ (accessed 10 July 2009).

35   Brown, 'Britain and Drugs: Doctors Say Cannabis Can Cure You, While Our Worst Crack War Erupts in London', *Independent*, 15 November 1997, https://bit.ly/3ysx8s1.

36   Ball, 'Cannabis Campaign: Legalize This Safe Drug, Says BMA', *Independent*, 16 November 1997, https://bit.ly/3L4rkaO.

37   'Cannabis: Should It Be Decriminalised?', *Independent On Sunday* debate, conference held 11 December 1997, https://www.ukcia.org/library/conf/11dec97debate.php.

38   Ibid.

39   Ibid.

40   Ibid.

41   Brown, 'Britain and Drugs'.

42   BMA, *The Therapeutic Uses of Cannabis*, 77.

43   Bevins, 'Lords Cannabis Inquiry', *Independent*, 11 February 1998, https://bit.ly/3N5Ca1W.

44   House of Lords Select Committee on Science and Technology, 'Introduction', in *Cannabis: The Scientific and Medical Evidence*, https://publications.parliament.uk/pa/ld199798/ldselect/ldsctech/151/15102.htm (accessed 20 July 2020).

45   Iversen, interview.

46   Lord Walton of Detchant, interview by Suzanne Taylor.

47   House of Lords Select Committee on Science and Technology, 'Evidence', in *Cannabis The Scientific and Medical Evidence*, v.

48   House of Lords Select Committee on Science and Technology, *Cannabis: The Scientific and Medical Evidence*, https://publications.parliament.uk/pa/ld199798/ldselect/ldsctech/151/15102.htm (accessed 20 June 2020).

49   Iverson, interview.

50   House of Lords Select Committee on Science and Technology, 'Oral Evidence from Griffith Edwards', in *Cannabis: The Scientific and Medical Evidence; Evidence*, 3.

51   House of Lords Select Committee on Science and Technology, 'Oral Evidence from Department of Health Witnesses', in *Cannabis: The Scientific and Medical Evidence; Evidence*, 44–59.

52   House of Lords Select Committee on Science and Technology, 'Oral Evidence from the Witnesses from the MRC', in *Cannabis: The Scientific and Medical Evidence; Evidence*, 147.

53   Lord Walton, interview.

54   House of Lords Select Committee on Science and Technology, 'Medical Use of Cannabis and Cannabinoids: Review of the Evidence', in *Cannabis: The Scientific and Medical Evidence*, http://publications.parliament.uk/pa/ld199798/ldselect/ldsctech/151/15107.htm#a13.

55   Lord Walton, interview.

56   House of Lords Select Committee on Science and Technology, 'Recommendations', in *Cannabis: The Scientific and Medical Evidence*,

http://publications.parliament.uk/pa/ld199798/ldselect/
ldsctech/151/15110.htm#a28.

57 Lord Walton, interview.

58 Robson and Guy, 'Clinical Studies of Cannabis-Based Medicines',
242–5.

59 House of Lords Select Committee on Science and Technology,
'Recommendations', in *Cannabis: The Scientific and Medical Evidence*,
http://www.parliament.the-stationery-office.co.uk/pa/ld199798/
ldselect/ldsctech/151/15110.htm#a28.

60 Ibid.

61 Secretary of State for Health, 'Government Reply to the Report of
the House of Lords Select Committee on Science and Technology,
Cannabis: The Scientific and Medical Evidence (9th Report, HL paper 151,
Session 1997–8)'.

62 Iversen, interview.

63 House of Lords debates, Cannabis: Select Committee Report,
3 December 1998 (181203-09), https://publications.parliament.uk/
pa/ld199899/ldhansrd/vo981203/text/81203-09.htm (accessed
10 July 2009).

64 Ibid.

65 Ibid.

66 Ibid.

67 Secretary of State for the Home Department, 'Government Reply to
the Report of the House of Lords Select Committee'.

68 Ibid.

69 Ashraf, 'UK Government Responds', 1,077.

70 Iversen, interview.

71 BMA, *BMA Calls for Active Research Effort to Produce New Cannabis-Based
Drugs but Says Crude Cannabis Is Unsuitable for Medical Use*, press
release, 11 November 1998; BBC, *Doctors Say No to Legalised Cannabis*,
BBC, 11 November 1998, http://bbc.in/3LDfEwe.

72 Lord Walton, interview.

73 Iversen, interview.

74 Ibid.

75 Robson, interview.

76 Lord Walton, interview.

77 Iversen, interview.

78 INCB, *Report of the INCB for 2003*.

79 Hamid Ghodse, interview by Suzanne Taylor and Virginia Berridge.

80 INCB, *Report of the INCB for 1998*.

81 Ghodse, interview.

82 Ibid.

83 'INCB Annual Report 1998', INCB press release (New York: United Nations, 1999).

84 INCB, *Report of the INCB for 1998*.

85 Ghodse, interview.

86 Interviews with Pertwee, Robson, Ziajack, and Notcutt.

87 The Police Foundation, *Drugs and the Law*.

88 Ibid.

89 Ibid.

90 Ibid.

91 Ibid.

92 Ibid.

93 Ibid.

94 Goodchild and Dillion, 'Government Ducks the Cannabis Debate', *Independent*, 7 July 2001, http://www.independent.co.uk/news/uk/this-britain/government-ducks-the-cannabis-debate-677095.html; BBC, 'Government Dismisses Landmark Drug Inquiry', *BBC*, 7 February 2001, https://bbc.in/3sSG3j7.

95 Travis, 'Straw Tries to Soften Rejection of Drug Report', *The Guardian*, 8 February 2001, http://www.guardian.co.uk/uk/2001/feb/08/drugsandalcohol.alantravis.

96 Home Affairs Select Committee, *Report of the Independent Inquiry into the Misuse of Drugs Act 1971, Drugs and the Law, Minutes of Evidence*.

97 BBC, 'Ministers Reject Drugs Law Overhaul', *BBC*, 7 February 2001, https://bbc.in/3NwcxaB.

98 House of Lords Science and Technology Committee, *Therapeutic Uses of Cannabis*, http:// publications.parliament.uk/pa/ld200001/ldselect/ldsctech/50/5001.htm.

99 House of Lords Science and Technology Committee, 'Therapeutic Uses of Cannabis', in *Therapeutic Uses of Cannabis*, http://publications.parliament.uk/pa/ld200001/ldselect/ldsctech/50/5002.htm.

100 Ibid.

101 Ibid.

102 Ibid.

103 BBC, 'Lords Back Cannabis Use', *BBC*, 22 March 2001, https://bbc.in/3GrY25z (accessed 10 July 2009).

104 Home Affairs Committee, Minutes of Evidence Taken before the Home Affairs Committee, Session 2001-02, on the Work of the Home Office, HC 302, Q. 5.

105 Home Affairs Select Committee, *The Government's Drugs Policy*.
106 Department of Health, *Government Response to the House of Lords Select Committee on Science and Technology's Report on the Therapeutic Uses of Cannabis*.
107 Ibid.
108 Ibid.
109 ACMD, *The Classification of Cannabis*.

CHAPTER SEVEN

1   Kaptchuk, 'Intentional Ignorance', 389–433; Doll, 'Controlled Trials', 1,217–20; D'Arcy Hart, 'A Change in Scientific Approach', 572–3; Oakley, 'Experimentation and Social Interventions', 1,239–42.
2   Matthews, *Quantification and the Quest*.
3   Cochrane, *Effectiveness and Efficiency*.
4   Meldrun, 'Departures from the Design'.
5   Toth, 'Clinical Trials in British Medicine'.
6   A proof-of-principle trial is a proof-of-concept trial rather than a drug licensing exercise.
7   Healy, *The Creation of Psychopharmacy*, 312.
8   Ibid., 322.
9   Notcutt, interview.
10   Anita Holdcroft, interview by Suzanne Taylor.
11   Holdcroft, interview.
12   Holdcroft *et al.*, 'Case Report: Pain Relief with Oral Cannabinoids in Familial Mediterranean Fever', 546–50.
13   Robson and Guy, 'Clinical Studies of Cannabis-Based Medicine'.
14   Anthony Moffat, quoted in Crowther *et al.*, *The Medicalization of Cannabis*.
15   Flyer for the event, Holdcroft's personal papers.
16   Holdcroft, interview.
17   Anthony Moffat, quoted in Crowther *et al.*, *The Medicalization of Cannabis*.
18   BMA, *The Therapeutic Uses of Cannabis*.
19   Moffat, *Society Welcomes Cannabis Research Findings*, press release, Royal Pharmaceutical Society, 11 November 1999, archived version (from 24 September 2006) available from https://bit.ly/3zVuewW.
20   House of Lords Select Committee on Science and Technology, 'Evidence', in *Cannabis: The Scientific and Medical Evidence*, 188.
21   Ibid.

22 Zajicek, interview.

23 Holdcroft, interview.

24 Ibid.

25 Zajicek, interview.

26 Ibid.

27 House of Lords Select Committee on Science and Technology, 'Evidence', in *Cannabis: The Scientific and Medical Evidence*, 144.

28 Holcroft, interview.

29 Zajicek, interview.

30 Ibid.

31 House of Lords Select Committee on Science and Technology, 'Evidence', in *Cannabis: The Scientific and Medical Evidence*, 173.

32 Holdcroft, interview.

33 Zajicek, interview.

34 Holdcroft, interview.

35 Zajicek, interview.

36 Ibid.

37 Ibid.

38 Ibid.

39 Ibid.

40 Holdcroft, interview.

41 Zajicek, interview.

42 Geoffrey Guy, quoted in Crowther *et al.*, *The Medicalization of Cannabis*.

43 House of Lords Select Committee on Science and Technology, 'Evidence', in *Cannabis: The Scientific and Medical Evidence*, 50.

44 Zajicek, interview.

45 ISRCTN control trials website, http://www.controlled-trials.com/ISRCTN25994117 (accessed 13 May 2009).

46 BBC, 'Cannabis May Be as Addictive as Cocaine', 16 October 2000, http://bbc.in/3lAdoeD; Clark, 'More Dangerous Than Heroin', *The Times*, 11 December 2002, https://www.thetimes.co.uk/article/more-dangerous-than-heroin-3c3dv5hvlcs (accessed 27 June 2022).

47 Holdcroft, interview.

48 Ibid.

49 Hall and Pacula, *Cannabis Use and Dependence*, 2.

50 Holdcroft, interview.

51 Ibid.

52 Ibid.

53 Ibid.

54   Ibid.

55   Holdcroft, Doré, and Maze, 'Cannabis in Postoperative Pain: A Dose Finding Study', 462.

56   Holdcroft *et al.*, 'A Multi-Centre Dose-Escalation Study', 1,040–6.

57   Zajicek, interview.

58   Ibid.

59   Ibid.

60   Ibid.

61   MHRA, *Public Information Report on Sativex Oromucosal Spray* (London: MHRA, 2006), archived version (from 17 February 2009) available from https://bit.ly/3O6VA7n.

62   Zajicek, interview.

63   Ibid.

64   MHRA, *Public Information Report on Sativex Oromucosal Spray.*

65   Metz and Page, 'Oral Cannabinoids for Spasticity in Multiple Sclerosis', 1,517–26.

66   Notcutt, 'Medicinal Cannabis Extracts in Chronic Pain', 26.

67   Robson, interview.

68   Zajicek, interview.

69   Ibid.

70   Ibid.

71   Ibid.

72   Ibid.

73   MRC, *MRC Funds Further Research To Look into the Role of Cannabis-Based Medicines in MS Treatment,* press release, 2003, http://www.mrc.ac.uk/Newspublications/News/MRC001902 (accessed 13 May 2009; URL no longer active).

74   Zajicek, interview.

75   Ibid.

76   Holdcroft, interview.

77   Zajicek, interview.

78   Zajicek, 'Lessons Learnt from the Cannabinoids MS (CAMS) Study', paper presented at the IACM Cannabis Symposium, Leiden, 9–10 September 2005.

79   Zajicek, interview.

80   Russo, *Cannabis: From Pariah to Prescription,* 3.

81   House of Lords Select Committee on Science and Technology, *Therapeutic Uses of Cannabis.*

82 Medicines Commission, Minutes of the Meeting Held on 13 May 2005, archived version (from 5 December 2014) available from https://bit.ly/3sTXBeq.

83 Iverson, *The Science of Marijuana.*

84 MS Society, MS *Society Dismayed at Latest* MHRA *Decision on Sativex,* press release, 10 June 2005, http://www.mssociety.org.uk/news_events/news/research/research_archive.html (URL no longer active).

85 Layward, interview.

86 Zajicek *et al.,* 'Cannabinoids for Treatment of Spasticity and Other Symptoms Related to Multiple Sclerosis', 1,517–26.

87 MS Society, *Cannabis Derived Medicine Can Improve Quality of Life* (London: MS Society, 2003), http://www.multsclerosis.org/news/Nov2003/CannabisDerivedMedicinesCanImproveQualityofLife.html (accessed 7 December 2019; URL no longer active).

88 MS Society, *Health Technology Appraisal: Cannabinoids for Symptom Relief in Multiple Sclerosis,* http://www.mssociety.org.uk/downloads/ACF5D9B.a340e54e.pdf (accessed December 2010; ULR no longer active as of July 2019).

89 Ibid.

90 Iverson, *The Science of Marijuana,* 136.

91 MHRA, *Sativex Appeal Decision,* press release, 10 June 2005, archived version (from 6 December 2014) available from https://bit.ly/3GfuKGR.

92 MHRA, *Importation of Sativex,* press release, 15 November 2005, archived version (from 6 December 2014) available from https://bit.ly/38OVstH.

93 GW Pharmaceuticals, *UK Named Patient Prescribing for Sativex,* press release, 15 November 2005, available from https://www.investegate.co.uk/gw-pharmaceuticals–gwp-/rns/re-sativex-update/200511150700401224U.

94 Holdcroft, interview.

95 MHRA, *Importation of Sativex.*

96 MHRA, *Public Information Report on Sativex Oromucosal.*

97 Ibid.

98 Ibid.

99 Griffith Edwards, quoted in Crowther *et al., The Medicalization of Cannabis.*

CHAPTER EIGHT

1   INCB, *Report of the INCB for 2019.*
2   Hall and Babor, 'Cannabis Use and Public Health', 488.
3   Murray, 'No Smoke without Fear', *The Guardian*, 17 September 2002, https://www.theguardian.com/lifeandstyle/2002/sep/17/healthandwellbeing.health1.
4   Johnston, 'UK "Too Soft on Cannabis Dangers"', *Telegraph*, 27 June 2006, http://www.telegraph.co.uk/news/uknews/1522399/UK-too-soft-on-cannabis-dangers.html.
5   ACMD, *Further Consideration of the Classification of Cannabis.*
6   House of Commons Science and Technology Committee, *Drug Classification: Making a Hash of It?*
7   Secretary of State for the Home Department, *The Government Reply to the Fifth Report from the House of Commons Science and Technology Committee, Session 2005–06 HC 1031, 'Drug Classification: Making a Hash of It?'.*
8   ACMD, *Cannabis: Classification and Public Health.*
9   House of Commons debates, 7 May 2008, vol. 475, col. 705, https://publications.parliament.uk/pa/cm200708/cmhansrd/cm080507/debtext/80507-0004.htm.
10 Tran, 'Government Drug Adviser David Nutt Sacked', *The Guardian*, 30 October 2009, https://www.theguardian.com/politics/2009/oct/30/drugs-adviser-david-nutt-sacked.
11 Hodges, quoted in Crowther *et al.*, *The Medicalization of Cannabis*, 69.
12 Sample, 'Cannabis: Scientists Call for Action amid Mental Health Concerns', *The Guardian*, 15 April 2016, https://www.theguardian.com/science/2016/apr/15/cannabis-scientists-call-for-action-amid-mental-health-concerns.
13 Power, 'Stoners Cheered When Canada Legalised Cannabis. How Did It Go So Wrong?', 5 April 2020, *The Guardian*, https://www.theguardian.com/society/2020/apr/05/stoners-cheered-when-canada-legalised-cannabis-how-did-it-all-go-wrong.
14 WHO, 'WHO Review of Cannabis and Cannabis-Related Substances', WHO website, https://www.who.int/teams/health-product-and-policy-standards/controlled-substances/who-review-of-cannabis-and-cannabis-related-substances.
15 WHO, Expert Committee on Drug Dependence, *Thirty-Ninth Report.*
16 CND, *CND Votes on Recommendations for Cannabis and Cannabis-Related Substances*, press release, 2 December 2020, https://bit.ly/3LBcusB.

17   BBC, 'Alfie Dingley "Amazingly Well" after Cannabis Treatment', *BBC*, 27 October 2018, https:// bbc.in/3sRY290.

18   Sajid Javid, Home Secretary Statement on Medical Use of Cannabis, Oral Statement to Parliament, 19 June 2018, https://www.gov.uk/ government/speeches/home-secretary-statement-on-medical-use-of-cannabis.

19   Simons, 'Jeremy Hunt Reveals He Backs Legalising Use of Medicinal Cannabis Oil', *Huffington Post*, 18 June 2018, https://bit. ly/3Njhgw8.

20   BBC, 'Medicinal Cannabis Products to Be Legalised', *BBC*, 26 July 2018, https:// bbc.in/3lD5IIA.

21   Sajid Javid, 'Rescheduling of Cannabis-Based Products for Medicinal Use', Statement UIN HCWS994, 11 October 2018, https://bit.ly/ 3LcGb36.

22   Schraer, 'Medicinal Cannabis: Why Has It Taken So Long to Get to Patients?', *BBC*, 16 February 2019, https://bbc.in/38foeUe.

23   Boseley, 'Watchdog Declines to Back NHS Cannabis Treatment for Epilepsy', *The Guardian*, 8 August 2019, https://www.theguardian. com/society/2019/aug/08/watchdog-declines-to-back-nhs-cannabis-treatment-for-epilepsy.

24   BMJ, 'Access to Medical Cannabis Must Be Improved, Argue Top Doctor and Mother of Alfie Dingley', *BMJ Newsroom*, 1 May 2019, https://www.bmj.com/company/newsroom/access-to-medical-cannabis-must-be-improved-argue-top-doctor-and-mother-of-alfie-dingley.

25   Health and Social Care Committee, *Drugs Policy: Medicinal Cannabis*, House of Commons report, HC 1821, 2019.

26   Mike Barens, quoted in Health and Social Care Committee, *Drugs Policy: Medicinal Cannabis*, point 41, https://publications.parliament.uk/pa/cm201719/cmselect/ cmhealth/1821/182106.htm.

27   NHS England and NHS Improvement, *Barriers to Accessing Cannabis-Based Products for Medicinal Use on NHS Prescription*, report, August 2019.

28   BMJ, 'Access to Medical Cannabis Must Be Improved'.

29   Burns, 'No government-funded medical cannabis clinical trials ongoing, two years since legalisation', *Pharmaceutical Journal*, 30 October 2020, https://pharmaceutical-journal.com/article/news/ no-government-funded-medical-cannabis-clinical-trials-ongoing-two-years-since-legalisation.

30 Health Europa, 'Cancard Launched Today', Health Europa website, 30 November 2020, https://www.healtheuropa.eu/cancard-uk-medical-cannabis-card-launched-today/104214.

31 Wilkson, 'GPS Warned Against Involvement in "Cancard" Cannabis ID Scheme', *Pulse*, 12 April 2021, https://www.pulsetoday.co.uk/news/clinical-areas/pain/gps-warned-against-involvement-in-cancard-cannabis-id-scheme.

32 Gornall, 'Big Cannabis in the UK'.

33 Adams, 'Legalising Cannabis Would Result in Soaring Numbers of People Suffering from Schizophrenia-Like Psychosis, One of Britain's Top Psychiatrists Has Warned', *Daily Mail*, 2 April 2020, https://www.dailymail.co.uk/news/article-8211293/Legalising-cannabis-result-people-suffering-psychosis.html.

34 Sharma, 'Brexit Stops "Life-Saving" Medical Cannabis Drug Supply for Epileptic Boy', *Independent*, 6 January 2021, https://www.independent.co.uk/news/uk/brexit-cannabis-drug-epileptic-netherlands-b1783012.html.

35 O'Carroll, 'Mother Fears Son Could Die as Brexit Stops Medical Cannabis Supply', *The Guardian*, 5 January 2021, https://www.theguardian.com/politics/2021/jan/05/mother-fears-son-could-die-as-brexit-stops-medical-cannabis-medicine-supply.

Bibliography

ARCHIVES CONSULTED

The National Archives (TNA), London.
Royal Pharmaceutical Society (RPS), London.
Wellcome Library, London.
World Health Organization (WHO), Geneva, Switzerland.

UK PARLIAMENTARY DEBATES

House of Commons debates (*Hansard*), 5th series, vol. 298; 6th series,
   vols. 163, 248, 263, 475, 595.
House of Lords debates (*Hansard*), 5th series, vol. 298.

INTERVIEWS

Flynn, Paul, by Suzanne Taylor, 14 August 2007.
Ghodse, Hamid, by Suzanne Taylor and Virginia Berridge, 22 February
   2008.
Hodges, Clare (Clare Brice), by Suzanne Taylor, 10 October 2007.
Holdcroft, Anita, by Suzanne Taylor, 2009.
Iverson, Leslie, by Suzanne Taylor, 30 August 2007.
Layward, Lorna, by Suzanne Taylor, 3 June 2009.
Lord Walton of Detchant, by Suzanne Taylor, 2007.
Mars, Sarah, by Virginia Berridge and Suzanne Taylor, 23 November
   2005.
Mechoulam, Raphael, by Suzanne Taylor, 2007.
Notcutt, William, by Suzanne Taylor, 2007.
Pertwee, Roger, by Suzanne Taylor, 24 August 2007.
Potter, David, by Suzanne Taylor, 23 July 2007.
Robson, Philip, by Suzanne Taylor, 28 June 2007.
Zajicek, John, by Suzanne Taylor, 9 November 2007.

PUBLISHED SOURCES

Abel, E. *Marihuana: The First Twelve Thousand Years.* New York: Plenum Press, 1980.

Abrams, J. *Science, Politics and the Pharmaceutical Industry.* London: UCL Press, 1995.

Abrams, S. 'Cannabis Law Reform in Britain'. In *The Marijuana Papers,* edited by D. Solomon, 69–79. London: Panther, 1969.

– 'The Wootton Report: The Decriminalisation of Cannabis in the UK'. DrugText website, 1997, http://www.drugtext.org/library/articles/WRaltnet.html.

Addiction Research Foundation and World Health Organization. *Report of an ARF/WHO Scientific Meeting on Adverse Health and Behavioral Consequences of Cannabis Use, Toronto, Ontario, 30 March–3 April, 1981.* Toronto: ARF, 1981.

Advisory Council on the Misuse of Drugs. *The Classification of Cannabis Under the Misuse of Drugs Act 1971.* London: The Stationery Office (TSO), 2002.

– *Further Consideration of the Classification of Cannabis under the Misuse of Drugs Act 1971.* London: TSO, 2005.

– *Cannabis: Classification and Public Health.* London: TSO, 2008.

Advisory Committee on Drug Dependence, Hallucinogens Sub-committee. *Cannabis: Report by the Advisory Committee on Drug Dependence.* London: TSO, 1968.

Aldrich, M. 'History of Therapeutic Cannabis'. In *Cannabis in Medical Practice: A Legal, Historical and Pharmacological Overview of the Therapeutic Use of Marijuana,* edited by M.L. Mathre, 35–55. London: Carload and Co., 1997.

Anderson, S., ed. *Making Medicines.* London: Pharmaceutical Press, 2005.

Arber, A. *Herbals: Their Origin and Evolution; A Chapter in the History of Botany, 1470–1670.* Cambridge: Cambridge University Press, 1986.

Ashraf, H. 'UK Government Responds to the Cannabis Debate'. *Lancet* 353, no. 9,158 (1999): 1077.

Ashton, C.H. *Cannabis: The Clinical and Pharmacological Aspects.* Department of Health Report for the ACMD, May 1998.

Asscher, W. 'Oral Evidence'. In *Therapeutic Uses of Cannabis,* by the House of Lords Select Committee on Science and Technology, 188. London: TSO, 2001.

Baker, D., G. Pryce, J.L. Croxford, P. Brown, R.G. Pertwee, J.W. Huffman, and L. Layward. 'Cannabinoids Control Spasticity and

Tremor in a Multiple Sclerosis Model'. *Nature* 404, no. 6,773 (2000): 84–7.

Barker, A., and B.G. Peters. *The Politics of Expert Advice: Creating, Using and Manipulating Scientific Knowledge for Public Policy.* Edinburgh: Edinburgh University Press, 1993.

Barnes, J. 'Therapeutic Applications of Cannabinoids'. Conference review of a meeting organised by the Pharmaceutical Sciences Group of the Royal Pharmaceutical Society of Great Britain and the Multiple Sclerosis (MS) Society of Great Britain and Northern Ireland, 1997, available from http://www.medicinescomplete.com/journals/fact/current/fact0203a17cr02.htm (URL no longer active; a copy is in the author's personal archive).

Barnes, P.J. 'Drugs for Asthma'. *British Journal of Pharmacology* 147 (2006): S297–303.

Basu, A.R. 'Cannabis and Madness: Evidence from the Indian Hemp Drugs Commission, Bengal, 1894'. *Studies in History* 16, no. 1 (2000): 131–8.

Berridge, V. *Opium and the People.* London: Allen Lane, 1981.

– 'Altered States: Opium and Tobacco Compared'. *Social Research* 68, no. 3 (2001): 656.

– 'Changing Places: Illicit Drugs, Medicines, Tobacco and Nicotine in the Nineteenth and Twentieth Centuries'. In *Biographies of Remedies: Drugs, Medicines and Contraceptives in Dutch and Anglo-American Healing Cultures,* edited by M. Gijswijt-Hofstra, G.M. van Heteren and E.M. Tansey, 11–34. Amsterdam: Rodopi, 2002.

– 'Queen Victoria's Cannabis Use: Or, How History Does and Does Not Get Used in Drug Policy-Making'. *Addiction Research and Theory* 11, no. 4 (2003): 213–15.

– *Marketing Health: Smoking and the Discourse of Public Health in Britain, 1945–2000.* Oxford: Oxford University Press, 2007.

Bewley-Taylor, D.R. *The United States and International Drug Control, 1909–1999.* London: Pinter, 1999.

– 'The Drugs Problem of the 1960s'. In *Heroin Addiction and the British System: Origins and Evolution,* edited by J. Strang and M. Gossop, 43. New York and London: Routledge, 2005.

Blech, J. *Inventing Diseases and Pushing Pills: Pharmaceutical Companies and the Medicalisation of Normal Life.* London: Routledge, 2006.

Bloomquist, E.R. *Marijuana.* Los Angeles, CA: Glencoe Press, 1968.

Bock, A. *Waiting to Inhale: The Politics of Medical Marijuana.* Santa Ana, CA: Seven Locks Press, 2000.

Bone, C., and S. Walden. 'New Trends in Illicit Cannabis Cultivation in the United Kingdom of Great Britain and Northern Ireland'. *Bulletin on Narcotics*, 49–50, no. 1 (1997), https://www.unodc.org/unodc/en/data-and-analysis/bulletin/bulletin_1997-01-01_1_page006.html.

Booth, M. *Cannabis: A History*. London: Doubleday, 2003.

British Medical Association. *The Misuse of Drugs*. Amsterdam: Harwood Academic Publishers, 1997.

– *The Therapeutic Uses of Cannabis*. Amsterdam: Harwood Academic, 1997.

Brunn, K., L. Pan, and I. Rexed. *The Gentlemen's Club: International Control of Drugs and Alcohol*. Chicago, IL: University of Chicago Press, 1975.

Brunner, T. 'Marijuana in Ancient Greece and Rome? The Literary Evidence'. *Bulletin of the History of Medicine* 47 (1973): 344–55.

Bulmer, M. 'The Royal Commission and Departmental Committee in the British Policy-Making Process'. In *Advising Western Governments*, edited by G. Peters and A. Barker, 37–49. Edinburgh: Edinburgh University Press, 1993.

'Cannabinoids for Nausea'. *Lancet* 317, no. 8,214 (1981): 255–6.

Carson, R. *Silent Spring*. London: Penguin Books, 1962.

Casto, D. 'Marijuana and the Assassins: An Etymological Investigation'. *International Journal of Addiction* 5, no. 4 (1970): 747–55.

Chang, A.E., D. Shilling, and R.C. Stillma. 'Delta-9-Tetrahydrocannabinol as an Antiemetic in Cancer Patients Receiving High-Dose Methotrexate'. *Annals of Internal Medicine* 91 (1979): 819–24.

Chawira, A., D.C. Warhurst, B.L. Robinson, and W. Peters. 'The Effect of Combination of Qinghaosu with Standard Antimalarial Drugs in the Suppressive Treatment of Malaria in Mice'. Transactions of The Royal Society of Tropical Medicine and Hygiene 81 (1987): 554–8.

Clark, A.R. 'Medical Aerosol Inhalers: Past, Present, and Future'. *Aerosol Science and Technology* 22, no. 4 (1995): 374–91.

Cochrane, A.L. *Effectiveness and Efficiency: Random Reflections on Health Services*. London: Nuffield Provincial Hospitals Trust, 1972.

Cohen, S. 'Therapeutic Aspects'. In *Marihuana Research Findings: 1976*, 194–214. NIDA Research Monograph 14. Washington, DC: US Government Publishing Office, 1976.

Commission on Narcotic Drugs. *The Question of Cannabis*. CND Resolution XII, 1957.

Concar, D. 'High Anxieties: What the WHO Doesn't Want You to Know about Cannabis'. *New Scientist*, issue 2,122, 1998.

Crowther, S.M., L. Reynolds, and T. Tansey. *The Medicalization of Cannabis: The Transcript of a Witness Seminar Held by the Wellcome Trust Centre for the History of Medicine at UCL, London, on 24 March 2009*. Wellcome Witnesses to Twentieth Century Medicine, no. 40. London: Wellcome Trust Centre for the History of Medicine, UCL, 2010.

D'Arcy Hart, P. 'A Change in Scientific Approach: From Alternation to Randomised Allocation in Clinical Trials in the 1940s'. *British Medical Journal* 319, no. 7,209 (1999): 572–3.

Davies, B.H., R.M. Weatherstone, and J.D.P. Graham. 'A Pilot Study of Orally Administered Delta Nine Trans THC in the Management of Patients Undergoing Radiotherapy for Carcinoma of the Bronchus'. *British Journal of Clinical Pharmacology* 1 (1974): 301–6.

Department of Health. *Government Response to the House of Lords Select Committee on Science and Technology's Report on the Therapeutic Uses of Cannabis.* London: TSO, 2001. Available from http://www.archive. official-documents.co.uk/document/cm53/5332/5332.pdf.

Devane, W., F. Dysarz, M. Johnson, L. Melvin, and A. Howlett. 'Determination and Characterization of a Cannabinoid Receptor in Rat Brain'. *Molecular Pharmaceutics* 34 (1988): 605–13.

Devane, W., L. Hanus, A. Breuer, R.G. Pertwee, L.A. Stevenson, G. Griffin, D. Gibson, A. Mandelbaum, A. Etinger, and R. Mechoulam. 'Isolation and Structure of a Brain Constitute that Binds to the Cannabinoid Receptor'. *Science* 258, no. 5,090 (1992): 1946–9.

Dobson, M. 'Bittersweet Solutions'. *Parasitologia* 40 (1998): 64–81.

Doll, R. 'Controlled Trials: The 1948 Watershed'. *British Medical Journal* 317, no. 7,167 (1998): 1217–20.

Dufton, E. *Grass Routes.* New York: Basic Books, 2017.

DuQuesne, J.T. 'Cannabis and the Rule of Law'. *Lancet* 318, no. 8,246 (1981): 581.

Economic and Social Council. *The Question of Cannabis: Medical Use of Cannabis Drugs (1959/730) (XXVIII).* New York: ESC, 1959.

Epstein, S. *Impure Science: AIDS, Activism and the Politics of Knowledge.* Berkeley and Los Angeles, CA: University of California Press, 1996.

Fairbairn, J.W., J.A. Liebmann, and S. Simic. 'The Tetrahydrocannabinol Content of Cannabis Leaf'. *Journal of Pharmacy and Pharmacology* 23, no. 7 (1971): 558–9.

Florin, D. *How Does Science Influence Policy? Health Promotion for Coronary Heart Disease by General Practitioners.* London: University of London Press, 1997.

– 'Scientific Uncertainty and the Role of Expert Advice: The Case of Health Checks for Coronary Heart Disease Prevention by General Practitioners in the UK'. *Social Science and Medicine* 49 (1999): 1269–83.

Gill, E.W., W.D.M. Paton, and R.G. Pertwee. 'Preliminary Experiments on the Chemistry and Pharmacology of Cannabis'. *Nature* 228, no. 5,267 (1970): 134–6.

– 'Propyl Homologue of Tetrahyrocabinol: Its Isolation from Cannabis, Properties and Synthesis'. *Journal of the Chemical Society* (1971): 579–82.

Glatt, M.M. 'Historical Note: Hashish and Alcohol "Scenes" in France and Great Britain 120 Years Ago'. *British Journal of Addiction to Alcohol and Other Drugs* 64, no. 1 (1969): 99–108.

Goode, E. 'Marijuana and the Politics of Reality'. *Journal of Health and Social Behaviour* 10, no. 2 (1969): 83–94.

Goodman, J., and V. Walsh. *The Story of Taxol.* Cambridge: Cambridge University Press, 2006.

Gornall, J. 'Big Cannabis in the UK: Is Industry Support for Wider Patient Access Motivated by Promises of Recreational Market Worth Billions?'. *British Medical Journal* 368 (2020): article m1002.

Graham, J.D.P. 'The 2-Halogenoalkylamines'. *Progress in Medicinal Chemistry* 2 (1962): 132–71.

– 'The Effect of Delta1-Tetrahydrocannabinol on the Uptake of [3H]-(minus)-Noradrenaline by the Isolated Perfused Heart of the Rat'. *British Journal of Pharmacology* 51, no. 3 (1974): 465–6.

– 'If Cannabis Were a New Drug'. In *Cannabis and Health,* 417–37. London: Academic Press, 1976.

– *Cannabis Now.* Aylesbury: HM&M Publishers, 1977.

– 'Cannabis and the Cardiovascular System'. *British Medical Journal* 1, no. 6,116 (1978): 857.

– 'The Bronchodilator Action of Cannabinoids'. In *Cannabinoids as Therapeutic Agents,* edited by R. Mechoulam. Boca Raton, FL: CRC Press, 1986.

Graham, J.D.P, and H. al Katib. 'The Action of Trypsin on Blockade by 2-Halogenoalkylamines: Speculation on the Nature of the Alpha Receptor for Catecholamine'. *British Journal of Pharmacology and Chemotherapy* 28 (1966): 1–14.

Graham, J.D.P., and G.W.L. James. 'The Pharmacology of a Series of Substituted 2-Halogenoalkylamines'. *Journal of Medicinal and Pharmaceutical Chemistry* 3 (1961): 489–504.

Graham, J.D.P, and D.M. Li. 'Cardiovascular and Respiratory Effects of Cannabis in Cat and Rat'. *British Journal of Pharmacology* 49 (1973): 1–10.

Guba, D.A. *Taming Cannabis: Drugs and Empire in Nineteenth-Century France.* Montreal and Kingston: McGill-Queen's University Press, 2020.

Guy, G. 'Introduction'. In *The Medicinal Uses of Cannabis and Cannabinoids*, edited by G. Guy, B. Whittle, and P. Robson, xxii. London: Pharmaceutical Press, 2004.

Guy, G., B. Whittle, and P. Robson, ed. *The Medicinal Uses of Cannabis and Cannabinoids*. London: Pharmaceutical Press, 2004.

GW Pharmaceuticals. 'Written Submission'. In *Cannabis: The Scientific and Medical Evidence; Evidence*, by the House of Lords Select Committee on Science and Technology, 160–73. London: TSO, 1998.

Hall, W., and T. Babor. 'Cannabis Use and Public Health: Assessing the Burden'. *Addiction* 95, no. 4 (2000): 488.

Hall, W., and R.L. Pacula. *Cannabis Use and Dependence: Public Health and Public Policy*. Cambridge: Cambridge University Press, 2003.

Hamlin, C. 'Expert Witnessing: Victorian Perspectives on a Modern Problem'. *Social Studies of Science* 16, no. 3 (1986), 485–513.

Hartley, J.P., S.G. Nogrady, and A. Seaton. 'Bronchodilator Effect of Delta1-Tetrahydrocannabinol'. *British Journal of Clinical Pharmacology* 5, no. 6 (1978): 523–5.

Healy, D. *The Creation of Psychopharmacology*. Cambridge, MA: Harvard University Press, 2002.

Hepler, R.S., I. Frank, and R. Petrus. 'Ocular Effect of Marijuana Smoking'. In *The Pharmacology of Marihuana*, edited by M.C. Braude, S.I. Szara, and the NIDA, vol. 2, 815–24. New York: Raven Press, 1976.

Herzberg, D. *White Market Drugs*. Chicago, IL: The University of Chicago Press, 2020.

Hilgartner, S. *Science on Stage: Expert Advice as Public Drama*. Redwood City, CA: Stanford University Press, 2000.

Hill, S. 'G-Protein-Coupled Receptors: Past, Present and Future'. *British Journal of Pharmacology* 147 (2006): S27–37.

Hill-Curth, L. *From Physick to Pharmacology: Five Hundred Years of British Drug Retailing*. Ashgate: Routledge, 2006.

Himmelstein, H. *The Strange Career of Marihuana: Politics and Ideology of Drug Control in America*. London: Greenwood, 1983.

Hindmarch, I. 'A Social History of the Use of Cannabis Sativa'. *Contemporary Review* 220 (1972): 252–7.

Holdcroft, A., C. Doré, and M. Maze. 'Cannabis in Postoperative Pain: A Dose Finding Study'. *British Journal of Anaesthesia* 91 (2003): 462.

Holdcroft, A., M. Maze, C. Doré, S. Tebbs, and S. Thompson. 'A Multi-Centre Dose-Escalation Study of the Analgesic and Adverse Effect of an Oral Cannabis Extract (Cannador) for Postoperative Pain Management'. *Anesthesiology* 104 (2006): 1040–6.

Holdcroft, A., M. Smith, A. Jacklin, H. Hodgson, B. Smith, M. Newton, and F. Evans. 'Case Report: Pain Relief with Oral Cannabinoids in Familial Mediterranean Fever'. *Anesthesia* 52 (1997): 483–8.

Holdcroft, A., M. Smith, B. Smith, H. Hodgson, and F. Evans. 'Clinical Trial Experience with Cannabinoids'. *Pharmaceutical Sciences* 3 (1997): 546–50.

Home Affairs Select Committee. *Report of the Independent Inquiry into the Misuse of Drugs Act 1971, Drugs and the Law, Minutes of Evidence.* HC 561-i 8, June 2000, http://www. publications.parliament.uk/pa/cm199900/cmselect/cmhaff/561/0060801.htm.

– Minutes of Evidence Taken before the Home Affairs Committee, Session 2001–02, on the Work of the Home Office. HC 302, Q. 5.

– *The Government's Drug Policy: Is It Working?* London: TSO, 2002. Available from http://www.publications.parliament.uk/pa/cm200102/cmselect/cmhaff/318/31808.htm.

Home Office. *Tackling Drugs to Build a Better Britain: The Government's Ten-Year Strategy for Tackling Drugs Misuse.* London: TSO, 1998.

– 'Written Submission'. In *Cannabis: The Scientific and Medical Evidence; Evidence,* by the House of Lords Select Committee on Science and Technology, 50. London: TSO, 1998.

Honigsbaum, M. *The Fever Trail.* London: Macmillan, 2001.

House of Commons Science and Technology Committee. *Drug Classification: Making a Hash of It?* London: TSO, 2006. Available from www.publications.parliament.uk/pa/ld199899/ldselect/ldsctech/39/3904.htm.

House of Lords Select Committee on Science and Technology. *Cannabis: The Scientific and Medical Evidence.* Ninth report for the session 1997–8. London: TSO, 1998.

– *Cannabis: The Scientific and Medical Evidence; Evidence.* London: TSO, 1998.

– *Therapeutic Uses of Cannabis.* Second report for the session 2000–1. London: TSO, 2001.

Hughes, J., T.W. Smith, H.W. Kosterlitz, L.A. Fothergill, B.A. Morgan, and H.R. Morris. 'Identification of Two Related Pentapeptides from the Brain with Potent Opiate Agonist Activity'. *Nature* 258 (1975): 577–9.

International Narcotics Control Board. *Report of the International Narcotics Control Board for 1998.* New York: United Nations, 1998.

– *Report of the International Narcotics Control Board for 2003.* New York: United Nations, 2003.

– *Report of the International Narcotics Control Board for 2019.* New York: United Nations, 2019.

International Union for Conservation of Nature, World Health
    Organization, and World Wildlife Fund International. *Guidelines on the
    Conservation of Medicinal Plants.* Gland, Switzerland: IUCN in partnership
    with WHO and WWF, 1993.
Iverson, L. *The Science of Marijuana*, 2nd ed., unpublished draft. Oxford:
    Oxford University Press.
Jasanoff, S. *The Fifth Branch: Science Advisers as Policymakers.* Cambridge,
    MA: Harvard University Press, 1990.
Kabelik, J. 'Hemp (*Cannabis sativa*): Antibiotic Drugs; I; Hemp in the Old
    and Popular Medicine'. *Pharmazie* 12, no. 7 (1957): 439–43.
Kalant, O. 'Ludlow on Cannabis: A Modern Look at a Nineteenth
    Century Drug Experience'. *International Journal of Addiction* 6, no. 2
    (1971): 309–22.
– 'Report of the Indian Hemp Drugs Commission, 1893–94: A Critical
    Review'. *International Journal of Addiction* 7, no. 1 (1972): 77–96.
Kaptchuk, T. 'Intentional Ignorance: A History of Blind Assessment and
    Placebo Controls in Medicine'. *Bulletin of the History of Medicine* 72, no. 3
    (1998): 389–433.
Kirby, C. 'Medicinal Plants and the Control of Protozoal Disease with
    Particular Reference to Malaria'. *Transactions of the Royal Society of
    Tropical Medicine and Hygiene* 90 (1996): 605–9.
Klawiter, M. *The Biopolitics of Breast Cancer: Changing Cultures of Disease and
    Activism.* Minneapolis, MN: University of Minnesota Press, 2008.
Klein, A., and G. Potter. 'The Three Betrayals of the Medical Cannabis
    Growing Activist: From Multiple Victimhood to Reconstruction,
    Redemption and Activism'. *International Journal of Drug Policy* 53 (2018):
    65–72.
Kosviner, A., D. Hawks, and M.G. Webb. 'Cannabis Use amongst British
    University Students: I; Prevalence Rates and Differences between
    Students Who Have Tried Cannabis and Those Who Have Never
    Tried It'. *British Journal of Addiction to Alcohol and Other Drugs* 69, no. 1
    (1974): 35–60.
Krejci, Z. 'Antibacterial Action of Cannabis Indica'. *Lek List* 7, no. 20
    (1952): 500.
– 'Hemp (*Cannabis sativa*): Antibiotic Drugs; II; Method and Results of
    Bacteriological Experiments and Preliminary Clinical Experience'.
    Pharmazie 13, no. 3 (1958): 155–66.
Lancet, The. 'The Therapeutic Possibilities in Cannabinoids'. Editorial.
    Lancet 305, no. 7,908 (1975): 667–9.
– [Gerard Vaughan (Minister of Health)?]. 'Government Policy on
    Cannabis'. *Lancet* 318, no. 8,246 (1981): 574.

Lewis, A. 'Historical Perspective'. *British Journal of Addiction to Alcohol and Other Drugs* 63, no. 3 (1968): 241–5.

Loewe, S. 'The Active Principles of Cannabis and the Pharmacology of the Cannabinols'. *Archiv fur Experimentale Pathologie und Pharmakologie* 211 (1950): 175–93.

Lorway, R. *AIDS Activism, Science and Community across Three Continents.* New York: Springer, 2017.

Lowy, I., and J.P. Gaudilliere. *The Invisible Industrialists: Manufacture and the Construction of Scientific Knowledge.* London: Macmillan, 1998.

MacLeod, R. *Public Science and Public Policy in Victorian England.* Brookfield, VT: Variorum, 1995.

Mathre, M. 'Cannabis Series: The Whole Story; Part 4; Research and Development of Cannabis Preparations and Delivery Systems'. *Drugs and Alcohol Today* 2, no. 2 (2002): 3–7.

– 'Cannabis Series: The Whole Story; Part 5; Research and Development of Cannabis Preparations and Delivery Systems'. *Drugs and Alcohol Today* 2, no. 4 (2002): 4–8.

– ed. *Cannabis in Medical Practice: A Legal, Historical and Pharmacological Overview of the Therapeutic Use of Marijuana.* London: Carload and Co., 1997.

Matthews, J.R. *Quantification and the Quest for Medical Certainty.* Princeton, NJ: Princeton University Press, 1995.

Matthews, P. *Cannabis Culture: A Journey Through Disputed Territory.* London: Bloomsbury, 1999.

McAllister, W. *Drug Diplomacy in the Twentieth Century: An International History.* New York and London: Routledge, 1999.

Mead, A. 'International Control of Cannabis: Changing Attitudes'. In *The Medicinal Use of Cannabis and Cannabinoids,* edited by G. Guy, B. Whittle, and P. Robson, 369–424. London: Pharmaceutical Press, 2004.

Mechoulam, R., ed. *Cannabinoids as Therapeutic Agents.* Boca Raton, FL: CRC Press, 1986.

Mechoulam, R., and E.A. Carlini. 'Towards Drugs Derived from Cannabis'. *Naturwissenschaften* 65, no. 4 (1978): 174–9.

Mechoulam, R., and Y. Gaoni. 'A Total Synthesis of dl-Delta-1-Tetrahydrocannabinol, the Active Constituent of Hashish'. *Journal of the American Chemical Society* 87 (1965): 3273–5.

Mechoulam, R., and L. Hanus. 'A Historical Overview of Chemical Research on Cannabinoids'. *Chemistry and Physics of Lipids* 108, no. 1–2 (2000): 1–13.

Meldrun, M. 'Departures from the Design: The Randomized Clinical Trial in Historical Context, 1946–1970'. Ph.D. Thesis, State University of New York, 1994.

Merlin, M. *Man and Marijuana: Some Aspects of their Ancient Relationship.* Rutherford, NJ: Associated University Press, 1972.

Metz, L., and S. Page. 'Oral Cannabinoids for Spasticity in Multiple Sclerosis: Will Attitudes Continue to Limit Use?'. *Lancet* 362, no. 9,395 (2003): 1517–26.

Mikuriya, T. 'Marijuana in Medicine: Past, Present and Future'. *California Medicine* 110, no. 1 (1969): 34–40.

Mills, J. *Madness, Cannabis and Colonialism: The 'Native-Only' Lunatic Asylums of British India, 1857–1900.* London: Macmillan, 2000.

– *Cannabis Britannica: Empire, Trade, and Prohibition, 1800–1928.* Oxford: Oxford University Press, 2003.

Mold, A. *Making the Patient-Consumer: Patient Organisations and Health Consumerism in Britain.* Manchester: Manchester University Press, 2015.

Multiple Sclerosis Society. *Health Technology Appraisal: Cannabinoids for Symptom Relief in Multiple Sclerosis.* Submission to the National Institute for Clinical Excellence (NICE), August 2003.

Musto, D. 'The 1937 Marijuana Tax Act'. *Archives Of General Psychiatry* 26, no. 2 (1972): 101–8.

Nahas, G. *Biomedical Aspects of Cannabis Usage.* New York: UNODC, 1977.

– *Keep off the Grass.* Exeter: A. Wheaton and Co., 1979.

Narrain, A., and V. Chandran. *Nothing to Fix: Medicalisation of Sexual Orientation and Gender Identity.* New Delhi: SAGE, 2016.

Newhart, M., and W. Dolphin. *The Medicalization of Marijuana.* New York and London: Routledge, 2019.

Nicolson, M., and G. Lowis. 'The Early History of the Multiple Sclerosis Society of Great Britain and Northern Ireland: A Socio-Historical Study of Lay/Practitioner Interaction in the Context of a Medical Charity'. *Medical History* 46, no. 2 (2002): 141–74.

Notcutt, W. 'Medicinal Cannabis Extracts in Chronic Pain: Comparison of Two Patients with MS'. Abstract, in *Congress of the IACM*, 26. Berlin: IACM, 2001.

Noyes, R. Jr., S.F. Brunk, D.A. Baram, and A. Carter. 'Analgesic Effect of Delta-9-Tetrahydrocannabinol'. *Journal of Clinical Pharmacology* 15, no. 2–3 (1975): 139–43.

– 'The Analgesic Properties of Delta-9Tetrahydrocannabinol'. *Clinical Pharmacology and Therapeutics* 18, no. 1 (1975): 84–9.

Oakley, A. 'Experimentation and Social Interventions: A Forgotten but Important History'. *British Medical Journal* 317, no. 7,167 (1998): 1239–42.

Organe, G., W.D.M. Paton, and E. Zamis. 'Preliminary Trials of Bistrimethylammonium Decane and Pentane Diiodide (C10 and C5) in Man'. *Lancet* 253, no. 6,540 (1949): 21–3.

Oudshoorn, N. 'United We Stand: The Pharmaceutical Industry, Laboratory, and Clinic in the Development of Sex Hormones into Scientific Drugs, 1920–1940'. *Science, Technology and Human Values* 18, no. 1 (1993), 5–24.

Paton, W.D.M. 'Drug Dependence: A Socio-Pharmacological Assessment'. *Advanced Science* 25, no. 124 (1968): 200–12.

– 'Drug Dependence: Pharmacological and Physiological Aspects'. *Journal of the Royal College of Physicians of London* 4, no. 3 (1970): 247–54.

– 'Pharmacology'. In *British Contributions to Medical Science*, edited by W. Gibson, 195–204. London: WIHM, 1971.

– 'Cannabis and Its Problems'. *Proceedings of the Royal Society of Medicine* 66, no. 7 (1973): 718–21.

– 'Cell Pathological Effects of Cannabis'. *Pharmaceutical Journal* 212 (1974): 340.

– 'The Contribution of Classical Pharmacological Methods to the Understanding of Psychoactive Drugs'. In *Animal Behaviour under the Influence of Psycho-Active Drugs: Proceedings of Conference at the National Institute of Public Health*, edited by J. van Noordwijk. Bilthoven: National Institute of Public Health, 1974.

– 'Molecular Basis of Drug Toxicity'. *Journal of Clinical Pathology* 28 (1975): 1–6.

– 'Additional Remarks on the Chronic Toxicity of Cannabis'. In *Cannabis and Related Drugs: The Significance of Medical and Experimental Work for the Formulation of Social Policy*, 105–24. Cambridge: Cambridge University Press, 1978.

– 'Achievements Resulting from Animal Research'. In *Biomedical Research Involving Animals: Proposed International Guiding Principles; Proceedings of the 17th CIOMS Round Table Conference*, edited by Z. Bankowski and N. Howard-Jones, 16–25. Geneva: WHO, 1983.

Paton, W.D.M., and R. Pertwee. 'The Actions of Cannabis in Man'. In *Marijuana: Chemistry, Pharmacology, Metabolism and Clinical Effects*, edited by R. Mechoulam, 287–333. London: Academic Press, 1973.

Paton, W.D.M., and D.M. Temple. 'Effects of Chronic and Acute Cannabis Treatment upon Thiopentane Anesthesia in Rabbits'. *Proceedings of the British Pharmacological Society* 44, no. 2 (1972): P346–7.

Perks, R., and A. Thomson, ed. *The Oral History Reader.* New York and London: Routledge, 2006.

Pertwee, R.G. 'The Ring Test: A Quantitative Method for Assessing the "Cataleptic" Effect of Cannabis in Mice'. *British Journal of Pharmacology* 46 (1972): 753–63.

– 'Cannabinoid Pharmacology: The First 66 Years'. *British Journal of Pharmacology* 147, supplement 1 (2006): S163–71.

Petersen C.R. *Marihuana Research Findings.* Rockville, MD: National Institute on Drug Abuse, 1977.

Pickstone, J. 'Medical Botany: Self-Help Medicine in Victorian England'. *Memoirs of the Manchester Literary and Philosophical Society, 1976–7* 119, (1977): 94–5.

Police Foundation. *Drugs and the Law: Report of the Independent Inquiry into the Misuse of Drugs Act 1971.* London: Police Foundation, 1999.

Potter, A., and D. Weinstock. *High Time: The Legalization and Regulation of Cannabis in Canada.* Montreal and Kingston: McGill-Queen's University Press, 2019.

Potter, D. 'Growth and Morphology of Medicinal Cannabis'. In *The Medicinal Uses of Cannabis and Cannabinoids,* edited by G. Guy, B. Whittle, and P. Robson. London: Pharmaceutical Press, 2004.

Powers, H. 'Drug Resistant Malaria: The Global Problem and the Thai Response'. In *Western Medicine as Contested Knowledge,* edited by A. Cunningham, 262–87. Manchester: Manchester University Press, 1997.

Quirke, V. 'From Alkaloids to Gene Therapy: A Brief History of Drug Discovery in the 20th Century'. In *Making Medicines: A Brief History of Pharmacy and Pharmaceuticals,* edited by S. Anderson, 177–201. London: Pharmaceutical Press, 2005.

– 'Collaboration in the Pharmaceutical Industry'. New York and London: Routledge, 2016

Raft, D., Gregg, J., Ghia, J., and Harris, L. 'Effects of Intravenous Tetrahydrocannabinol on Experimental and Surgical Pain'. *Clinical Pharmacology and Therapeutics* 21, no. 1 (1977): 26–33.

Randall, R. 'Glaucoma: A Patient's View'. In *Cannabis in Medical Practice: A Legal, Historical and Pharmacological Overview of the Therapeutic Use of Marijuana,* edited by M. Mathre, 94–102. London: McFarland and Co., 1997.

Rang, H.P. 'The Receptor Concept: Pharmacology's Big Idea'. *British Journal of Pharmacology* 147 (2006): S9–16.

Robson, P. 'Therapeutic Aspects of Cannabis and Cannabinoids'. *British Journal of Psychiatry* 178 (2001): 107–15.

Robson, P., and G. Guy. 'Clinical Studies of Cannabis-Based Medicines'. In *The Medicinal Uses of Cannabis and Cannabinoids*, edited by G. Guy, B. Whittle, and P. Robson. London: Pharmaceutical Press, 2004.

Room, R., B. Fischer, S. Lenton, and W.D. Hall. *Cannabis Policy: Moving Beyond Stalemate*. Oxford: Oxford University Press/Beckley Foundation Press, 2010.

Rose, M. 'Cannabis: A Medical Question?'. *Lancet* 315, no. 8,170 (1980): 703.

– 'Cannabis and the Rule of Law'. *Lancet* 318, no. 8,238 (1981): 138.

Royal Pharmaceutical Society. 'Written Evidence'. In *Cannabis: The Scientific and Medical Evidence; Evidence*, by the House of Lords Select Committee on Science and Technology. London: TSO, 1998.

Russo, E. *Cannabis: From Pariah to Prescription*. London: Haworth Press, 2003.

– 'History of Cannabis as a Medicine'. In *The Medicinal Use of Cannabis and Cannabinoids*, edited by G. Guy, B. Whittle, and P. Robson. London: Pharmaceutical Press, 2004.

Sallan, S.E., N.E. Zinberg, and E. Frei. 'Antiemetic Effect of Delta-9-THC in Patients Receiving Cancer Chemotherapy'. *New England Journal of Medicine* 293 (1975): 795–7.

Saper, A. 'The Making of Policy Through Myth, Fantasy and Historical Accident: The Making of America's Narcotics Laws'. *British Journal of Addiction to Alcohol and Other Drugs* 69, no. 2 (1974): 183–93.

Schultes, R., and S. von Reis. *Ethnobotany: Evolution of a Discipline*. London: Chapman and Hall, 1995.

Secretary of State for Health. 'Government Reply to the Report of the House of Lords Select Committee on Science and Technology, *Cannabis: The Scientific and Medical Evidence* (9th Report, HL paper 151, session 1997–1998)'. Appendix 2 in the second report of the House of Lords Select Committee on Science and Technology for the session 1998–99, https://bit.ly/3FxIZXo.

– *Government Reply to the Fifth Report from the House of Commons Science and Technology Committee, Session 2005-06 HC 1031, 'Drug Classification: Making a Hash of It?'*. London: TSO, 2006. Available from https://assets.publishing.service.gov.uk/government/uploads/system/uploads/attachment_data/file/272360/6941.pdf.

Sherratt, A. 'Peculiar Substances'. In *Consuming Habits: Drugs in History and Anthropology*, edited by J. Goodman, P. Lovejoy, and A. Sherratt, 1–10. New York and London: Routledge, 1995.

Shiva, V. *Biopiracy*. Totnes, UK: Green Books, 1998.

Slinn, J. 'Research and Development in the UK Pharmaceutical Industry from the Nineteenth Century to the 1960s'. In *Drugs and Narcotics in History*, edited by R. Porter and M. Teich, 168–86. Cambridge: Cambridge University Press, 1995.

– 'The Development of the Pharmaceutical Industry'. In *Making Medicines: A Brief History of Pharmacy and Pharmaceuticals*, edited by S. Anderson, 155–74. London: Pharmaceutical Press, 2005.

Solomon, D. ed. *The Marijuana Papers*. London: Panther, 1969.

Society for Mental Awareness. 'The Law Against Marijuana is Immoral in Principle and Unworkable in Practice'. Advertisement, *The Times*, 24 July 1967.

Spriggs, T.L.B. 'J.D.P. Graham'. *British Journal of Pharmacology* 99, no. 1 (1990): 3–4.

Star, S., and J. Griesemer. 'Institutional Ecology, "Translations" and Boundary Objects: Amateurs and Professionals in Berkeley's Museum of Vertebrate Zoology, 1907–39'. *Social Studies of Science* 19, no. 3 (1989): 387–420.

Strang, J., and M. Gossop. *Heroin Addiction and the British System: Origins and Evolution*. New York and London: Routledge, 2005.

Tansey, E.M., D.A. Christie, and L.A. Reynolds. 'Drugs in Psychiatric Practice'. In *Wellcome Witnesses to Twentieth Century Medicine: Witness Seminar Transcripts*, edited by E.M. Tansey, D.A. Christie, and L.A. Reynolds. London: Wellcome Trust, 1998.

Taylor, S.L., and V. Berridge. 'Medicinal Plants for the Control and Treatment of Infectious Tropical Disease: A Case Study of Research at the London School of Hygiene and Tropical Medicine, 1899–2000'. *Transactions of the Royal Society of Tropical Medicine and Hygiene* 100 (2006): 707–14.

Toth, B. 'Clinical Trials in British Medicine, 1858–1948, with Special Reference to the Development of the Randomised Controlled Trial'. Ph.D. Thesis, University of Bristol, 1998.

Trace, M., A. Klein, and M. Roberts. *Reclassification of Cannabis in the United Kingdom*. DrugScope Briefing Paper 1, The Beckley Foundation Drug Policy Programme. London: DrugScope, 2004.

Tylden, E., and W.D.M. Paton. 'Clinical Aspects of Cannabis Action'. In *Marijuana*, edited by R. Mechoulam, 362. New York: Academic Press, 1973.

Ungerleider, J.T., and T. Andrysiak. 'Bias and the Cannabis Researcher'. *Journal of Clinical Pharmacology* 21, supplement (1981): S153–8.

Ungerleider, J.T., T. Andrysiak, L. Fairbanks, G.W. Ellison, and L.W. Myers. 'Delta-9-THC in the Treatment of Spasticity Associated with Multiple Sclerosis'. *Advances in Alcohol and Substance Abuse* 7, no. 1 (1987): 39–50.

United Nations Information Service. *US Supreme Court Decision on Cannabis Upholds International Law.* INCB Press Release. New York: UNIS, 2003.

– *Marijuana Vending Machines in Los Angeles are Contrary to International Drug Control Treaties, Says INCB.* INCB Press Release. New York: UNIS, 2008.

Vicari, S., and F. Cappai. 'Health Activism and the Logic of Connective Action: A Case Study of Rare Disease Patient Organisations'. *Information, Communication and Society* 19, no. 11 (2016): 1653–71.

Weatherall, M. *In Search of a Cure: History of Pharmaceutical Discovery.* Oxford: Oxford University Press, 1990.

Werner, C.A. 'Medical Marijuana and the AIDS Crisis'. New York and London: Routledge, 2002.

Whittle, B., and G. Guy. 'Development of Cannabis-Based Medicine: Risks, Benefits and Serendipity'. In *The Medicinal Uses of Cannabis and Cannabinoids,* edited by G. Guy, B. Whittle, and P. Robson, 436. London: Pharmaceutical Press, 2004.

Williams, S.J., J.P. Hartley, and J.D.P. Graham. 'Bronchodilator Effect of Delta1-Tetrahydrocannabinol Administered by Aerosol of Asthmatic Patients'. *Thorax* 6, no. 31 (1976): 720–3.

Witton, J., S. Mars, and DrugScope. *Cannabis and the Gateway Hypothesis.* London: DrugScope, 2001.

Wood, B. *Patient Power? The Politics of Patient Associations in Britain and America.* Buckingham: Open University Press, 2000.

Woodcock, J. 'Cannabis Now'. *Health Education Journal* 37, no. 4 (1978): 248.

World Health Organization. *The Physical and Mental Effects of Cannabis.* Geneva: WHO, 1955.

– *The Use of Cannabis: Report by the WHO Scientific Group.* Geneva: WHO, 1972.

– *Traditional Medicine and Modern Health Care.* Document TRM/MTP/87.1. A44/10. Geneva: WHO, 1991.

– *Cannabis: A Health Perspective and Research Agenda.* Geneva: WHO, 1997.

World Health Organization, Expert Committee on Addiction-Producing Drugs. *Thirteenth Report.* Geneva: WHO, 1964.

World Health Organization, Expert Committee on Drug Dependence. *Seventeenth Report.* Geneva: WHO, 1970.

– *Eighteenth Report.* Geneva: WHO, 1970.

– *Nineteenth Report.* Geneva: WHO, 1972.
– *Twenty-Second Report.* Geneva: WHO, 1985.
– *Twenty-Third Report.* Geneva: WHO, 1987.
– *Twenty-Fourth Report.* Geneva: WHO, 1988.
– *Twenty-Fifth Report.* Geneva: WHO, 1989.
– *Twenty-Sixth Report.* Geneva: WHO, 1989.
– *Twenty-Seventh Report.* Geneva: WHO, 1991.
– *Twenty-Eighth Report.* Geneva: WHO 1993.
– *Thirty-Ninth Report.* Geneva: WHO, 2018.
World Health Organization, Expert Committee on Drugs Liable to
   Produce Addiction. *Report on the Second Session.* Geneva: WHO, 1950.
– *Third Report.* Technical Report 57. Geneva: WHO, 1952.
Zajicek, J., P. Fox, H. Sanders, D. Wright, J. Vickery, A. Nunn,
   A. Thompson, and the UK Multiple Sclerosis Research Group.
   'Cannabinoids for Treatment of Spasticity and Other Symptoms
   Related to MS (CAMS study)'. *Lancet* 362 (2003): 1517–26.
– 'Lessons Learnt from the Cannabinoids in MS (CAMS) Study'. Paper
   presented at the IACM Cannabis Symposium, Leiden, 9–10 September
   2005.
Zarhin, Dana. 'The Trajectory of "Medical Cannabis" in Israel: Driving
   Medicalization in Different Directions'. *International Journal of Drug
   Policy* 82 (2020): article 102809.
Zarhin, Dana, Maya Negev, Simon Vulfsons, and Sharon R. Sznitman.
   '"Medical Cannabis" as a Contested Medicine: Fighting Over
   Epistemology and Morality'. *Science, Technology and Human Values* 45,
   no. 3 (2019): 488–514.

Index